Fat Chance

Fat Chance

My life in ups, downs and crisp sandwiches

LOUISE McSHARRY

PENGUIN
IRELAND

PENGUIN IRELAND

UK | USA | Canada | Ireland | Australia
India | New Zealand | South Africa

Penguin Ireland is part of the Penguin Random House group of companies
whose addresses can be found at global.penguinrandomhouse.com.

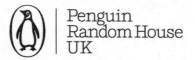

First published 2016
001

To protect people's privacy, some names and identifying details of non-family members have been changed

Set in 13.5/16pt Garamond MT Std
Typeset by Palimpsest Book Production Limited, Falkirk, Stirlingshire
Printed in Great Britain by Clays Ltd, St Ives plc

A CIP catalogue record for this book is available from the British Library

ISBN : 978–1–844–88370–7

www.greenpenguin.co.uk

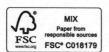

Penguin Random House is committed to a
sustainable future for our business, our readers
and our planet. This book is made from Forest
Stewardship Council® certified paper.

For my family,
who managed to buck untraditional beginnings to
become completely mental – in a very normal way

Contents

Preface

There's nothing like your wedding day to make you take stock. Although it's a beginning, it can feel a bit like an ending, too. On my wedding day, 21 August 2015, I certainly found myself looking back.

If you're lucky, everyone you love is at your wedding. I had chosen the room I was going to get ready in especially so I could see everyone arriving (though they couldn't see me). I had set up shop in front of the window with my make-up bag (top tip: You gotta have some natural light when you're doing your make-up). I had given myself an hour to apply it slowly and carefully while at the same time checking out our families and friends and what they were wearing. It was my very own private *This is Your Life*.

There were my grandparents, who had given me some of the safest, most beautiful moments of my childhood. There was my dad, walking around like he was running the show, his pacing betraying some of his excitement and nerves. There were my aunt and uncle, Greg and Linda, who had supported me through my most difficult and insecure teenage days. There were my new in-laws, who had shown me what it would be like to be part of a drama-free family. There was my biological mother, Dee, with whom I have the most difficult relationship in my life, but I was really grateful that she was there. There was another of my aunts, wearing . . . oh my God! . . . *the same dress as my mom*.

Once the panic over the dress mess had died down (my

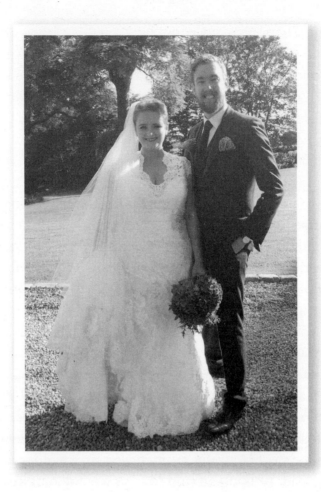

mom ran straight up the stairs to me for advice, and we agreed she had no choice but to change into the dress she had chosen for the following day), I turned my attention to the film crew, where the producer of a documentary was waiting to ask me some questions. That was another thing that made me look back in wonder: I had a camera crew at my wedding. RTÉ was making a TV documentary about me having had cancer.

Cancer. I still find that hard to believe.

I'd been working with Aoife, the producer, for the previous year. She wanted to know how I felt about cancer now that I was out the other side of it. I heard myself saying that, in a way, cancer had become a friend to me. I was surprised at this, but at the time I really felt that way. In a weird way, cancer and I had been through something together. The year just gone had been such a journey of growth and experience I couldn't hate the thing that had started it.

That sense of how much I had changed in a year was never clearer to me than the moment I put on my wedding dress. Of course, I had thoughts about my body and its size. The voices in my head that wished I were smaller were not silent. However, cancer gave me another voice: *How amazing it is to be getting into this dress, feeling as well as I do. Hasn't my body served me well?*

The day carried on in that vein. I looked back, but I also lived joyously in the moment. *Yes, I have been through a lot. But look at me now. Look at all I've learned. Look where I am. Look how lucky I am.*

Lucky. It's a funny word. Not one I used to think I would use to describe my life. It just goes to show, if you are somehow open to it, luck can come your way despite the circumstances. Because, on the face of it, I got some unlucky breaks in life.

Things got off to a rough start for me. That's not a complaint, it's just a fact.

My father, Winston, who I remember very little of, died when I was three. He was twenty-eight and, after having spent some years in remission, the cancer he had first been diagnosed with at eighteen took his life. It's sad he died so young. It's sad he left behind two infant children. It's sad he died worrying about his wife's drinking.

My mother, Dee, is an incredible woman, and when she

3

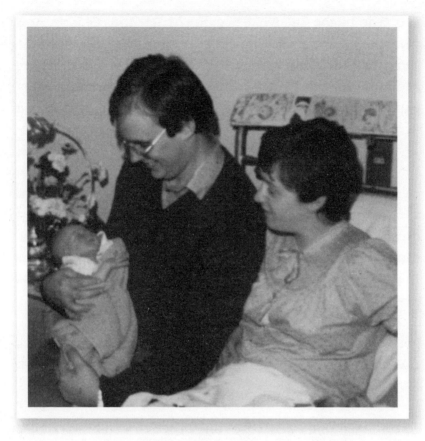

Day 1. With my father and mother, Winston and Dee Merriman.

was sober she was an incredible parent. Sadly, she wasn't sober enough of the time, and the drinking that had disturbed my dad when he was dying became a much bigger problem afterwards. So when he died, I also lost a normal childhood.

By the time I was seven I had taken on the role of parent, both to my younger brother, Andrew, and to Dee. I put Andrew to bed and distracted him when we were living in a house full of alcoholics and drug addicts. I poured Dee's vodka down the sink while begging her to stop drinking. And when it all came to a head and the authorities got involved I lied to the nice lady who wanted to know if we were happy and well taken care of, even though I was wearing filthy clothes and we were living in squalor. Maintaining an image of normality had become my most important job.

The level of responsibility I took on while still a child is sometimes difficult for me to get my head around now. It is extremely difficult for Dee to think about, too. She's sober now, after years and years of drinking and losing everything except her life to it. The 'what if' thoughts plague her. What if things had been different? What if she'd been able to be a mother?

I shared those thoughts for a long time. I missed her, desperately, and as I got older I always felt like something was missing. Like something was wrong with me. I was not a popular girl: I did not have the right clothes and, as I was constantly reminded by kids at school, I was fat.

Inevitably, I hit a few bumpy patches along the way as I grew up and became an adult. Stupid promiscuity, because I didn't care enough about myself. Ups and downs in work, particularly the trauma of being dumped from a job I loved (worse than cancer, believe it or not). Being fat – that's always been a big deal. And then, just as everything was on track and I was sorted and planning to marry the love of my life, I got cancer.

You know what? I wouldn't change a thing. Because – brace yourself for the cliché – it has all been the making of me, just as all of your experiences have been the making of you. Someday, you may find yourself in a situation

Someday, you may find yourself in a situation where someone asks you, 'How did you get through it?' This book is my answer to that question.

where someone asks you, 'How did you get through it?' This book is my answer to that question.

The other thing about a life with a lot of drama is that all the ordinary, mundane living has to get done in between. Getting up, getting dressed, eating, going to school, work. Friendships, falling out of friendships, crushes. In between the big, scary stuff that was going on I discovered all the things that could give me a lift: make-up and music and friends; falling into a profession I absolutely love; falling in love with someone who also fell in love with me . . . So while there's a lot in this book about how I got through the hard times, there's also lots here about all the stuff I love, and the stuff I don't love so much but that made me what I am. It's more or less how I got to thirty-three in eight chapters of pain, fun, sex, love, embarrassment, joy, achievement, stupidity, pride, effort, doubt, war paint, crisps, confidence and courage.

1
Growing up

Barbie Ferrari . . .
and what might have been

I am three and my family is gathered in the sitting room surrounded by presents, with the lights on. The sky outside is
grey, and my parents are yawning. My dad, in fact, is lying on
the couch in his dressing gown because he is well into his
second run-in with cancer. We don't know it, but it is one of
the last times he will come downstairs. In my mind's eye, I
pretend he is lying on the couch just because he is tired and
I'd woken him up at the crack of dawn, like your typical child
on your typical Christmas morning.

And like your typical child on a typical Christmas morning, I
was fixated on one thing only: my present. I had been dreaming
of a Barbie Ferrari for what felt like months, and I couldn't
really imagine a world in which Santa Claus hadn't brought me
one. When the wrapped box was put in front of me I must have
been like a rabid dog, ripping it apart. Sure enough, there it was,
my very own Barbie Ferrari. I'd love to tell you it was a thing of
beauty but, in truth, the 80s wasn't a great decade for car design.
Nonetheless, I adored that dull, angular contraption. I insisted
on getting it out of the box as quickly as possible, which was
about forty minutes, given all the bloody twisty-ties on every bit
of every Barbie thing ever produced. But I couldn't believe it: it
was all mine. My very own designer car.

Still sitting in the detritus of wrapping paper, cardboard
and twisty-ties, I began to roll the Ferrari along the ground,
imagining how chic my Barbies were going to look in it later
that day and what outfits they'd be wearing.

And then my brother vomited in it.

He hadn't been around for long, my brother, but I had adjusted to him. In many ways, he had become my favourite person. I liked his smiley face and how 'taking care of him' made me feel grown up. However, on this occasion, if I could have killed him I would have. I was hysterical. There's no other word for it. I wailed and wailed as my mother attempted to clean it up, my father laughing at the scene. Soon my mother was laughing, too, an injustice I felt to my very core. I don't remember much of what happened next, just that I never played with that Barbie Ferrari again. I was convinced I could smell the baby sick on it, and the shine had well and truly gone off it. Also, I was never able to let go of the sense of injustice that, in my time of need, my parents had chosen to laugh at me.

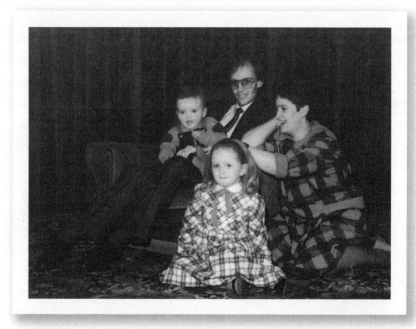

The complete Merriman family, December 1985 —
Winston, Dee, baby Andrew and me.

That Christmas morning has become one of my favourite memories, injustice and all. The reason is simple. Not only is that my first memory, it is also my last memory of feeling like I was part of a normal family. Not long after that, my father died. The alcoholism that was in my mother already now took over her life, and toys slid down the list of my priorities as I took on adult responsibilities at ages five, six and seven.

While I'm able to look back at that morning with a feeling of warmth, it also makes me sad, because it is a picture of what might have been. What if my father hadn't died? Would we have been a happy, healthy family? To be honest, I doubt it. I think the drinking would have taken over my mother no matter what, and who knows what effect that would have had on us.

What if my father hadn't died? Would we have been a happy, healthy family?

I'm sorry to say that I haven't spent a huge amount of time thinking about my father. I don't have very many memories of Winston, and people tend not to speak about him around me. The gist I have always got is that he was a bit of an Abba-listening, plane-watching nerd. My favourite story about him came from my Uncle David, who told me about a morning when my father burst into his bedroom, knelt on David's chest and punched him in the face until he named every member of his favourite football team, Bohemians. Okay, it's a little violent, but at least it displays a spark of personality. A few months ago, I walked to the house they grew up in, around the corner from Dalymount (home of Bohs), and stood in front of it for a while. I gazed at the house, picturing that scene and straining to feel a connection to him.

It didn't really happen that day, but during my cancer

experience I did feel more of a connection with him. I felt that we finally had something in common. We both had cancer. We both had chemo. I wondered how he felt during his treatment. What his first thoughts after his diagnosis had been. How he had coped when it became clear he was going to die. When I was told my cancer was gone, I counted my lucky stars but felt sad that he had not been so lucky.

My first true feeling of emotion about him came around that time, when my grand-aunt Joan gave me a load of old photographs. She had decided to divide them up into piles for me and my cousins (presumably afraid that they would otherwise end up in the dump when she died; ever practical, Joan!). Every image in my envelope included me. It was amazing to see photographs from my early life in Ireland. The house of my paternal grandparents, the Merrimans, is plastered in pictures of all of us grandchildren, but to see a true glimpse of what my life was like before we moved to America was really moving.

One photo, in particular, got me going. It was taken in the house my father grew up in, and all of his brothers and sisters are in it, as well as my granny, my parents and me. My father is sick. You can tell from his gaunt face. His cheekbones are like razorblades, and he is almost unrecognizable as the same man holding an infant me in another photograph in the envelope. It's frightening. However, he is also happy and, sitting at his feet, freshly bathed and in pyjamas, is a tiny little me. His hands are tangled in my hair. It is one of the few photographs I have in which we are touching.

I struggled not to cry when I looked at it for the first time, and I am crying now, thinking about it. My tears are for him, for the life he could have had, and for the life he lost. My tears are also for me, for the life I could have had, and for the life I lost. A life where you know exactly where you come within

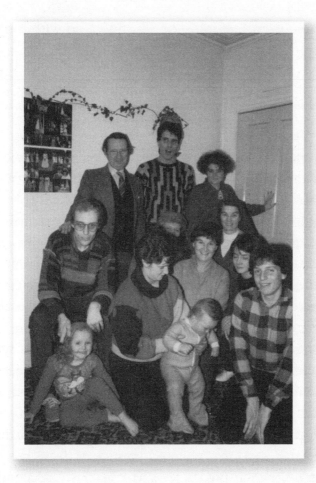

your family and one where you are confident of your connections. One where you can look back at photos of your father with his hands in your hair and reassure yourself that 'Yeah, he loves me.' One where people don't congratulate your parents for having 'taken them on', as though you and your brother are a burden, which, although you have surely brought your adoptive parents joy, you know you must have been at times. As much as I love the parents who raised me, and as happy as I am with where I am now, I don't think I will ever fully get over the sense of the loss of a 'normal' childhood.

Dee

You know how, every once in a while in Dublin, we have a perfect day. The clouds disappear and the sun shines and we tell each other what a great country it'd be 'if we only had the weather'. People pile out of their offices early to take advantage of the opportunity to enjoy a pint outside, kids in wetsuits dive into the canal, supermarkets sell out of burgers and the entire country smells like a barbecue. Your worries disappear and you feel an inexplicable sense of joy. Well, on days like these, I always feel compelled to listen to Paul Simon's *Graceland*.

The guitar riffs and harmonies transport me back to one of the truly perfect memories I have of my life with Dee. Judging by the release date of the album, I was four or five, and I remember sitting in the back of a red car we had won in a raffle. The windows, covered in stickers from our trip to Disneyland, were rolled down, and even the wind as we drove wasn't strong enough to prevent the heat of the sun warming my little face. Dee was driving and singing along, and I think we were on our way to the blood bank, in Dun Laoghaire, of all places. The sea was sparkling alongside us as we travelled, and I felt safe and happy. Dee was in a good patch.

There were many good patches, really. I'm not sure what prompted them. Sometimes they followed a stint in a treatment centre. Perhaps they occasionally followed a particularly scary episode of drinking during which she knew she had endangered us. I'm sure one followed the intervention my family, our neighbours and her GP had with her in our sitting room in Palmerstown while I sat pulling the wings from the dead flies on the windowsill.

I sometimes wonder if the good patches did us more harm than good. It's hard to give up on someone when they keep tempting you with how things could be. Hope can be a terrible thing.

> *It's hard to give up on someone when they keep tempting you with how things could be. Hope can be a terrible thing.*

It's really when I think about what things might have been like if Dee hadn't been an alcoholic that it gets sad. Because it probably would have been great. Without the booze, Dee was an amazing mother. She was fun, playful and loving. She told us she loved us all the time. I never doubted her, not for a minute. She adored me, was so proud of me and always made sure I looked the part of the adored bonny princess. And the evidence is the cover of this book – that is a picture of two-year-old me that appeared on the cover of *Woman's Way* when I was Ireland's Baby of the Year in 1984. While on bed rest during her pregnancy with my brother, Dee had entered me into the competition on a whim. She, Winston and I were also featured on the front of the *Evening Press* the day of the announcement.

I have so many lovely memories of Dee, from her lovingly brushing and plaiting my long hair in the morning to us cosying up on the couch and watching a film on a rainy day. She made up games for us to play, took out our favourite videos and made us tomato soup when we were sick. She taught me to love prawn cocktail and pâté and, over several hours on a sunny afternoon, how to blow a bubble with my chewing gum. She held a surprise birthday party for a little

Little Louise—a beauty queen already!

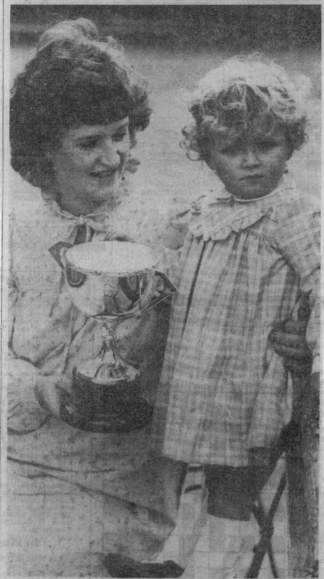

A BEAUTY Queen who punches her mum, slops her food and makes eyes at the boys is blonde blue - eyed Louise Merriman of Dublin, seen above with her mother Deirdre.

And during her year's reign she may do as she pleases because . . . she is onll 23 months old !

Chosen as the Heinz-Woman's Way Baby of the Yar, she received a silver trophy and a cheque for £250 from Mr. John P. O'Reilly, Chief Executive of Erin Foods yesterday at a special ceremony in the Dublin Zoo.

Unaware of the importance of her prize she wasn't even told she had entered the competition !

(Picture Matt Walsh) (See full story, Page Six.

Irish Independent

girl across the road when her family wasn't able to one year. When she got Andrew a BMX for Christmas, she stayed up half the night wrapping it. It wasn't in a box . . . she wrapped the actual bike. Every inch of it was covered.

She read to me and taught me to love books, joining in my excitement when I woke her up in the middle of the night to tell her that I had completed *Charlie and the Chocolate Factory* all on my own. When I was six she brought me to London and told me all about its history. When I figured out the truth about Santa and confronted her about it after bath-time one night, she admitted that I was right, hugging me in my towel and telling me how important it was to let other children hold on to believing in him for as long as possible.

One day when I was having a lovely time with her in front of the fire I felt so safe and loved I couldn't handle the immense guilt I was feeling over having stolen a two-pence piece from someone's coat in the cloakroom at school. The circumstance I found myself in was so lovely that I felt a bold girl like myself didn't deserve it. Dee told me I needed to go into school and tell the teacher what I'd done and give the two pence back. She also hugged me and told me she loved me. When she was good, she was oh so good.

By the time I was six, I'd been woken up in the middle of the night by my mother loads of times. Some of the memories are charming, like that scene in *Gilmore Girls* where Lorelai wakes up Rory to show her that it's snowing outside. But most of the time it was less storybook, more nightmare. Dee had moments of excitement so intense she simply couldn't let me sleep through them. Of course, she would be drunk as well.

On one occasion the vodka, and what I can only assume was mania, told her we should move to America. Not that we should apply for visas, sell our house and say goodbye to our family, but that we should go to the airport immediately and get on the next plane.

She came into my bedroom to wake me up with the news that we were leaving, grabbing my sleepy three-year-old brother as well. Andrew's little eyes struggled to stay open as we sat in the sitting room and she filled us in on the plan. She was in a panic because we were apparently going to miss our flight and instructed me to 'call the airport to tell the plane to wait'! I picked up the phone and pretended to have a conversation with someone at the airport, then reassured her that it was sorted. I knew enough to go along with the scenario and that it would run its course. In fact, I don't remember feeling scared at all.

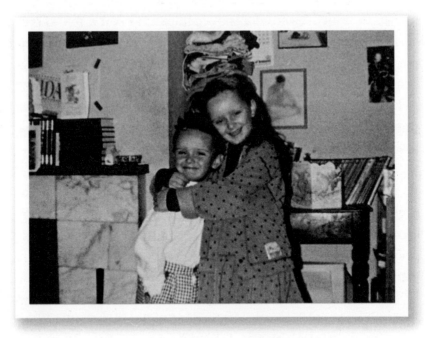

Andrew and I not long before we emigrated to America.
He's four and I'm seven.

Dee bundled us into our coats and out the front door into the quiet of our estate, keys jangling as she attempted to unlock the car in the dark. She struggled for a bit to get the key in the lock. Then she got the door open and we climbed in. I'm not sure what happened next. Perhaps she had a moment of clarity and realized that she shouldn't drive, or perhaps she had just worn herself out, but she never started the car. We waited in the back seat and, once she had fallen asleep, I climbed into the front, took the keys out of the ignition and brought Andrew into the house, leaving the door on the latch. The next morning she greeted us with a bright smile. Everything was back to normal.

Dee must have felt excruciating shame on mornings like the one after the airport incident, or any of the times a member of the bar staff was forced to ring someone to collect us from a pub where she was drinking. It really is no wonder that, when I drank from her orange juice at breakfast, it tasted bitter.

I got to know the taste of alcohol. I have so many memories of picking up her glass of Coke or orange juice, sipping from it and recognizing the taste. I don't remember being conscious of it then, but it seems obvious to me now that I was checking on her. Checking to see what kind of day it was going to be. I remember a moment when she saw me do it and our eyes met. I can still see her face then, her blue eyes full of sadness. She knew I knew. And I did know what was going on: I may have been six, but my feelings were those of an adult.

Though I stood at the sink pouring alcohol down the drain countless times – sometimes when Dee wasn't looking, other times while she shouted at me to stop, half laughing, half crying – at the same time, outside of the house, I was keen to pretend that all was well at home. If people asked about her, whether she was drinking or not, I would lie sweetly, batting my pretty eyelashes at them and deftly changing the subject.

Whether it was true or not, I felt like I was the glue holding our very fragile situation together.

> **Whether it was true or not, I felt like I was the glue holding our very fragile situation together.**

Things at home might have been inconsistent, but we had lots of support around us. We had amazing neighbours, the kind I'm not sure exist any more. More often than not we were out exploring the estate or playing on the green, but if I wasn't outside I could be in one of five houses on the road. We banged pots and pans outside our houses at midnight on New Year's Eve and gathered for annual photos in our bin-bag Hallowe'en costumes in October. Sometimes, if Dee was going through a rough patch, I would stay in our neighbour Theresa's house, and she would do everything within her power to make sure I wasn't aware of any of the drama that was going on. I'll never forget the good she did for me, or take it for granted. Our drama became her drama, and I'm sure she took on more worry than was fair.

Aside from the lovely people on our road, there was also family. My Granny Frances, Dee's mother, was a formidable woman. She worked as a physio until she was sixty-six, stopping only when they forced her to. She was sarcastic and loved a good slagging, both of herself and of others. She was always there for us and ensured that Andrew and I felt supported. At the same time, she never molly-coddled Dee over her drinking.

Most of Dee's brothers and sisters lived abroad but they also supported us in every way possible. I always felt loved.

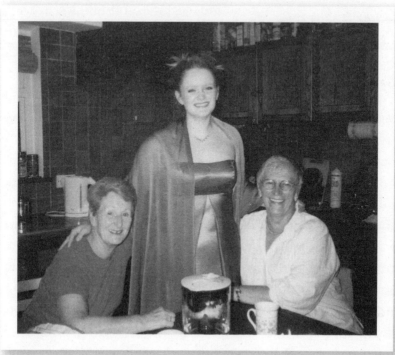

With my two grannies, Frances McSharry and Connie Merriman, the night of my debs, 2001.

Perhaps the greatest source of stability in those years, however, were my granny and grandad on my dad's side. They were entirely committed to our well-being and collected us every Sunday, without fail, to go and spend the day with them. We used to go on all kinds of adventures. Grandad loved to teach Andrew about his one true passion – trains – and Granny did her best to pass on her love of flowers to me. (I do love flowers, but let's just say I don't have a green thumb.) We would spend days at the seaside in the summer and go and look at the Christmas lights in the winter. They worked hard to make sure that we maintained relationships with that side of the family, taking us to visit our aunts and uncles and grand-aunts and great-grandparents. Things never felt more normal than when we were with them, and many of my favourite memories from those first seven years of my life are of times spent with them. The weekends always wrapped up with me in their sitting room in front of a special small table, eating a delicious crisp sandwich and watching something lovely on telly (ideally, the Dolly Parton show – that woman has owned my heart for almost thirty years).

The effort my grandparents took to care for us is something that still makes me emotional to this day. They managed to put on a sunny front for the two of us, but behind the scenes they were extremely worried. They did everything they could to protect us, seeking legal counsel in an attempt to have us go and live with them and staging interventions with Dee in attempts to get her well.

What it's like to have an alcoholic parent

If you want to know what it's like to have an alcoholic parent – here are some of the things you'll experience:

- Getting out of the car in the middle of nowhere because they've collected you from your friend's house and you've realized that they're drunk
- Repeatedly being called a bitch for questioning their behaviour
- Being told you'll ruin their marriage if you tell on them
- Dreading sports games and other school events because you can never be sure they won't turn up drunk
- Pitying glances
- Shredded pride
- An unending feeling of responsibility for them and for the rest of your family, though you are a child
- Making pathetic attempts to win their approval and be 'good enough' so that they'll stop drinking
- Pouring drink down the sink
- Cowering in corners
- Screaming matches
- Police cars in the driveway
- Fear every time you put your key in the front door
- Pleading with your other parent to leave them
- Christmases destroyed
- Waking up in the morning and genuinely puzzling over how they could be so drunk *already*
- Constant hope that they'll stop drinking
- Constant disappointment
- Lies to your face
- Constant pretence to the outside world

America

I was six and sitting in the kitchen eating my cereal one morning when Dee came into the kitchen, waving a letter. 'We got them!' she shouted. She was talking about Donnelly visas. It was the first I was hearing of it but, apparently, we were actually moving to America. She was excited. I remember feeling a faint sense of foreboding but didn't take her announcement too seriously. She was always coming up with big ideas, and they didn't always come to anything.

As it turned out, she was serious this time. Her plan was that we would move to Los Angeles, where she would start nursing again and we would all live happily ever after. She put our house on the market, we moved into a rented house . . . and then Dee really fell off the wagon. Away from bothersome family and neighbours, she would meet up with a drinking buddy and go into town. She was drunk all the time, and any semblance of keeping it together went out the window.

On my seventh birthday we woke up in her friend's house. It was the first of my birthdays on which I didn't wake up to Dee's happy face. Instead, I called her name up the stairs and she came hurtling down, trying to get it together, shouting 'Happy birthday!' with forced jollity. I remember the look in her eyes. She knew she was a mess. I knew she was a mess. But we both pretended everything was fine. This carried on for the duration of our final days in Ireland.

Behind the scenes, no one was happy about our move. My

father's parents did everything within their power to stop us going, but the solicitors advised them that they hadn't a hope of getting custody of us when we were with our biological mother. I can only imagine the fear our friends and family felt about our departure, especially considering Dee's drinking at the time. She must have been scared, but off we went on a cold day in November 1989, waving goodbye to the only life we'd ever known.

On our way to LA we stopped in Chicago to spend Christmas with her brothers. We stayed with Ruaidhrí and Ger, Dee's brother and his wife. They lived in a two-bedroom apartment and did their best to make us feel comfortable and welcome. I'm not sure how they did it, but they managed to talk Dee out of moving on to LA and, instead, she found us an apartment near them. We were enrolled in school and set about making our new lives.

It didn't take long for Dee to find people to socialize with in the way she liked to socialize. Our downstairs neighbours and their friends seemed happy to accommodate her drinking. So, she got back to her old habits. I vividly remember standing in the kitchen of our small apartment, pouring vodka down the sink – again – as she told me I was being silly . . . again. I was crying. She was crying.

It sounds grim, and it was, but I do also have some fond memories of Dee at that time. One day we each had to bring a hundred of something into school. I forgot mine and was in a blind panic, and then Dee showed up, to the rescue, having run to the school with a hundred strands of spaghetti. Around this time, she also taught me about racism. I'd never met anyone who wasn't white until we moved to America and she explained that what people looked like on the outside didn't matter because, on the inside, we all looked the same. We went to see

The Little Mermaid at the cinema. We ate soup together and watched *The Mickey Mouse Club* on TV after school. This was always the thing about Dee, and I think the thing that still devastates her. Dee had it in her to be an absolutely amazing mother. If it weren't for the drink. But there was always the drink.

> **Dee had it in her to be an absolutely amazing mother. If it weren't for the drink. But there was always the drink.**

Due to her innate charm, Dee never seemed to have any trouble getting a man, and she acquired a boyfriend in America in no time. His name was Tony, and he lived in a caravan by the river in a nearby town. I never liked him. I felt like he considered Andrew and me a nuisance but, even worse, I found him frightening. He used to make me watch him play with a knife. He'd throw it into a tree by his caravan at night-time, lit only by a bonfire. My suspicions that he was a bad guy were confirmed when he had the bright idea to rob a gun shop, at gunpoint, in daylight, while we were waiting for him in the car outside. Needless to say, he wasn't successful and we watched as he was led out of the shop in handcuffs. Dee was inconsolable. I was terrified. It's strange that, of all the things which happened over the years, this event is the one that sticks out as being particularly traumatic. I didn't like Tony, but still I found the idea of him being arrested and put in jail horribly upsetting. That situation brought home to me that our lives had really changed. I was no longer precious, safe in the hands of neighbours and grandparents. We were on our own now. I was really and truly scared.

While Tony was in prison, Dee hung out with a group of people she had met at one of his court appearances. They seemed to congregate in a house in Aurora, a nearby town. We sometimes spent our nights there. It was a party house. Everyone was drinking all the time. I know there were drugs there, too. Andrew and I used to hang around in the garage with one of the guys who owned the house. He and his older brother had inherited it from their parents, I think, and he didn't seem as into the scene as his brother. He spent most of his time working on cars but would go to the local fast-food restaurants to get us something to eat. I don't know if we would have eaten if it hadn't been for him.

I hated it in that house. I had an overwhelming sense that we just didn't belong there, and I hated the people I was surrounded by. One night, one of the people who lived in the house wept in front of me and told me it was because she couldn't see her children any more. It occurred to me that it could happen to us, too.

Tony got out of jail and Dee was excited to have him back. She wanted to be with him all the time and so she practically moved us into his caravan. We slept there night after night in our clothes, me wetting the bed each time and air-drying the bedclothes during the day. There was no plumbing, so no way of washing. We were filthy and hungry, surviving on uncooked hot dogs.

Meanwhile, the principal of my school was in touch with the local office of the Department of Children and Family Services about me. I hadn't been to school for weeks, and I can only assume there had already been some concerns because soon he had teamed up with Ruaidhrí and Ger to try to find us. Ruaidhrí spent his days cycling around the area in the hopes of figuring out where we were. Eventually, he spotted us.

The next day, a woman from the DCFS rapped on the door of the caravan. When it opened, she looked around in disgust. She needed to speak to us, but 'not here'. It was decided that we would meet her in her office a couple of hours later. Dee went into panic mode. We raced back to our apartment (why we had been living in the caravan when we still had an apartment is beyond me), where Dee bathed us and put us in our best clothes. When we arrived at the DCFS, we were back to our normal selves. We were the gorgeous, well-dressed children we had been in Ireland. But by then it was too late.

Andrew and I sat in an office with the woman who had rapped on the caravan door as she questioned us on what our lives were like. Andrew said very little. He had just turned five (he doesn't really remember much of this). I lied through my teeth. I knew what was going on, and I wasn't going to give anything away. It didn't make any difference, though. When we walked out of her office I turned to look towards the waiting area, where Dee was standing with her back to me. I could tell she was crying and I knew it was over.

We were ushered into a small room, where Ruaidhrí and Ger were waiting for us. Andrew sat with Ruaidhrí and made paper aeroplanes while I sat on Ger's lap and cried. The walls of the room were painted a cheerful yellow, and I felt like even that was mocking me. The jig was up. We were saying goodbye to Dee.

Ruaidhrí and Ger were granted temporary custody of us that day. For years, I thought we had been taken from Dee, but it turned out she surrendered custody. I'm proud of her for making that decision. As agonizing as it must have been at the time, she couldn't take care of us and it was for our own good that she admitted it.

Initially, there was still contact with Dee. At first our visits were supervised but after a while we got to see her on our own. However, it became clear that we couldn't rely on her to show up to these arranged visits. Contact dwindled. We never knew when we would hear from her. It might be a drunken phone call or a basket of presents on our front porch.

Sometimes she'd go through a really good spell. At times like that she made it difficult for me to give up on the fantasy of having my family back. At one stage she was working in a local café for months, beloved by customers and staff alike. Ger would take us there after school for something to eat so that we could see her and talk to her. Dee was the picture of health, sparkling and charismatic, telling me how beautiful I was – something I really needed to hear – and it was impossible not to feel a glimmer of hope that perhaps this was it, perhaps this was the time she was going to do it. Then the inevitable came. We went to visit one day only to find that she didn't work there any more. Her departure had been abrupt and unpleasant. We didn't go to the café any more. She was drinking again. Again.

The periods of absence were excruciating. All the while, all I really wanted was to be back with Dee in our familiar situation, toxic as it had been. For six years after we left her I spent every evening gazing out of my bedroom window, whispering, 'Star light, star bright, first star I see tonight, I wish I may, I wish I might, go back to living with my mom.' I blew out candles wishing with all my being that we could be together again. Slowly but surely, though, the constant disappointment became too much, and I suppose I gave up on her.

Anyone who knows an addict will be familiar with this. With having your heart broken, over and over again. In fact, I can imagine it will sound familiar to an addict, too. I can't think that Dee didn't feel the same level of disappointment as me every time she fell off the wagon; in fact, I suspect she felt it so badly she couldn't live

Anyone who knows an addict will be familiar with this. With having your heart broken, over and over again.

with it and poured herself another drink to numb the pain. The feeling of 'what if' is hard to shake, and it was not until six years after we went to live with Ruaidhrí and Ger that I decided I was done with her. That was the day she humiliated me in front of my friends. But that's a story for later.

It's hard for me to think about how grim things must have been for her during these years. I have never doubted her love for us, which I'm thankful for. I have always appreciated that, for her, alcoholism was not a choice. People who don't have any understanding of addiction tend to think: *How could you choose alcohol or drugs over your children?* I don't think it's that simple. By definition, being addicted means you *can't* stop doing the thing you're addicted to. I don't think she really had a choice at that time, because, if she had, she would have chosen us. I know that.

Nobody wants to be an addict. Nobody wants to have their life destroyed by a dependence on a substance. Nobody says, 'I want to be an addict when I grow up.' Largely, addiction is a symptom of a trauma. Addiction happens as a result of some dark experience in a person's life. That's why it kills me that so many people are so keen to look down their noses at people whose lives have been taken over by dependency.

If you're not an addict, count your lucky stars. Count your lucky stars that your life has not driven you to a darkness that is intolerable. Count your lucky stars that your circumstances haven't resulted in you growing up in a house which taught you that drinking and using drugs is the way to live. Thank your lucky stars, because there but for the grace of God go you.

Mean girls

The worst break-up of my life took place in 1996. I was thirteen, and her name was Shannen Walsh. We had been together for five years, having first connected in fourth grade. When we met I was still very much reeling from the big life changes that had happened over the last few years. I had emigrated, been adopted (by Ruaidhrí and Ger) and got a new surname and a new baby sister, changed schools and moved house three times over the space of eighteen months. I may have been eight, but I felt like I was thirty-five. Similarly, my adoptive parents – only in their twenties – were still adjusting to the new little people in their lives, both emotionally and financially. As a result of all this, I was not exactly a 'cool girl'. I didn't have the right clothes or school bag. I didn't do the right after-school activities. I didn't have the right accent. According to one girl's parents, I didn't even live in the right part of town. (That one really burned.)

However, none of that seemed to bother Shannen too much. She was a pretty, funny, confident girl, and we clicked in the classroom straight away. We became inseparable in the way that only girls can be. We spent all day at school together laughing at our own private jokes and writing each other notes. At each other's house we made up plays and dance routines. During sleepovers we would 'pretend to be kids', setting up fake shops with a real cash register someone had given her. We idolized her cheerleading older sister, Donna. In the later years, we spent hours learning the lyrics to 'Gangsta's Paradise', skipping

32

and pausing the CD over the course of half an hour to carefully write down the lyrics. When Shannen got the lead in our fifth-grade play, the part I wanted, I did my best to look happy for her. When the same thing happened in sixth grade, I found it a little more difficult: Shannen had everything I wanted, and my true, pure love for her was equalled only by intense envy.

Shannen had everything I wanted, and my true, pure love for her was equalled only by intense envy.

The biggest challenge we faced came in seventh grade, as we entered our teenage years. By then, our roles were clear. She was the cute, funny one, and I was her friend. There was a revolving cast of guys who fancied her, and therefore a revolving cast of guys who called me after school to talk about her. I answered their calls enthusiastically. If I couldn't have what I wanted myself, at least I could be near to it. We spent hours talking about the guys we liked, me nursing obsession after obsession over any guy who looked in my direction, she actually enjoying mini-relationships with the guys she liked. Frequently, the guys she went out with were guys I fancied, but I knew the part I had to play. That wasn't for the likes of me. I was happy for her. Most of the time.

One day we were on our way home on the school bus when her sister Donna deigned to speak to us. This was an extremely rare occurrence. Donna was two years older than us and, as well as her cheerleading prowess, she was beautiful and really and truly popular. She barely acknowledged our existence in her house, let alone in public. On this day, the bus was sparsely populated and she must have been bored because she decided to spark up a conversation. 'So, who do you guys like?' she asked, American parlance for 'Who do you fancy?'

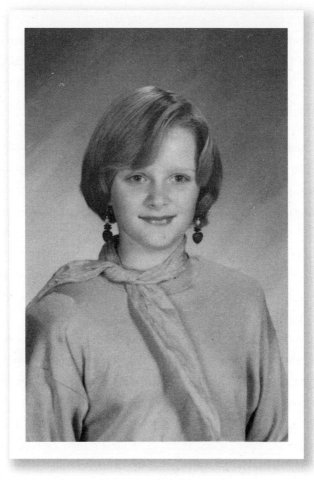

Aged eleven and dressing like the
35-year-old I thought I was.

Shannen, as keen to impress as I was, blurted out, 'Louise likes Steve Emerson!'

A hand – mine – flew out and slapped her across the face.

I couldn't believe I had done it. It happened so quickly, it felt like a truly involuntary action. Donna cuddled Shannen to her as she started to cry and looked at me as if I were a monster. 'I . . . I . . .' I could barely speak but managed to apologize repeatedly as we approached our bus stop. 'I'm so sorry, Shannen . . . I'm so, so sorry.' Donna glared at me and pulled her sister away as we got off the bus, and I was left standing at the corner in shock. How could I have done such a thing? Shannen was my best friend! I loved her!

When I got home I was too ashamed to say anything to my parents and, without Shannen, I had no one to talk to. The shame I felt was intense, and I arrived at school the next day filled with dread. When Shannen came in, her cheek and eye were black and blue. I had given her a black eye. *I had given her a black eye!* I couldn't believe it. She turned her head the other way as she passed me, and I ate my lunch in the toilets that day and for several days afterwards. I was mortified and ashamed, and felt absolutely distraught at being exiled from her life. We were rehearsing for the school play and I would gaze at her yearningly from a distance as she laughed with the other members of the cast. (It was *Robin Hood* and she was playing Maid Marian. Ahead of the auditions I had spent two weeks learning and rehearsing the role. But that was just the way things went – Shannen in a lead role and me in a bit part, playing an old lady.)

After a few weeks of utter misery, I happened to be in hospital for some tests, one of which required me to have a general anaesthetic. When I came to I was still a little loopy, and it was at this point that I revealed all to my mother. I laughed as I told her, 'I punched Shannen.' Over and over again I said it, first laughing and then dissolving into tears. My mother was horrified but sympathized with me. When we got home she phoned Shannen's mother to apologize.

Back at school Shannen seemed to defrost a little, and at

last she agreed to speak to me. I grovelled and she graciously accepted my apology. Clearly, she had been given approval to remain friends with me. We got back to normal and we had a further year and a half of true friendship.

Every year my parents did their best to cobble together enough money for us to get home to Ireland. Generally, we would stay for about six weeks, migrating from the house of one set of relatives to the next once we'd exhausted our welcome. I mostly loved it, especially the time spent with my cousins on the beach in Wexford and hanging out with my coolest aunt and uncle in their house. Upon my return each year, I would dash from the car to the house, grabbing the phone and dialling Shannen's number. 'I'm home! Want to come over?' Our reunions were always jubilant, the time spent apart evaporating as we struggled to tell each other the stories from our summer fast enough. At least, that was the case until the summer of 1996.

That year, I launched myself out of the car and towards the phone, as per usual, but when Shannen picked up she didn't sound like her usual self.

'D'you wanna come over?' I asked.

'Um . . . I have plans,' she said.

'Oh . . . okay,' I said, trying to hide my disappointment. She knew I was due home that day, so why had she made plans? 'What are you doing?'

She told me she was going to the cinema with three girls from school. They weren't girls we'd ever hung around with, and I felt a little nervous as I asked her if I could join them.

'I don't know if there's room in the car,' she said, and then – reluctantly – agreed that I could tag along. When I hopped into the car that evening the reception was frosty. I was in no doubt that her new friends were unhappy about my presence, and I could sense Shannen's unspoken apology during the short journey.

That was the beginning of the end. I tried to hang around with them but I wasn't wanted. When we started high school a couple of weeks later Shannen did everything she could to put space between us. I didn't realize how bad things were until one day in September when I found myself walking home, alone, with Sammy, one of the three girls. Sammy was the nicest one and somehow over the course of the journey she realized that I was not so bad and began to feel guilty about the way things had been going. She blurted out that a phone call I'd received the day before from Gina, the queen bee of the group, had not been as innocent as it might have seemed. I'd sensed that something was off. Gina wasn't in the habit of calling me and the conversation had felt more like an interview than anything else. She had questioned me about my feelings for Shannen, asking me repeatedly if I was annoyed with her and if I thought she was a bitch. I had replied nervously that I wasn't, and I didn't. Then the conversation had ended abruptly. If you've seen the film *Mean Girls* (and if you haven't, then I don't know what you're doing reading this book: you should go and watch it immediately), you'll know what's coming next. Yep, Shannen had been on the phone as well. Gina had rung me with the sole intention of luring me into speaking badly of Shannen. Sammy had been listening in, too.

I tried to react coolly, assuring Sammy that I had known all along. Inside, my heart was breaking. After we parted ways I ran the rest of the way home and made a beeline for the phone. Shannen didn't deny it. Our friendship was over.

I can honestly say that it was the most difficult break-up of my life. I couldn't understand it at all. I didn't know what I'd done or what had changed. How could it be that this person, who had been virtually my partner in life for years, now wanted nothing to do with me?

As an adult, I understand that, at that age, everything is changing. You're supposed to be figuring out who you are, and it seemed that while I was away Shannen had

How could it be that this person, who had been virtually my partner in life for years, now wanted nothing to do with me?

figured out that she wanted to be more like her new friends. When I came back she was probably confronted with the person she had been – a slightly goofier, less cool, less grown-up version of herself – and she didn't like it.

For my part, it seems obvious that, while I loved Shannen, I also despised her for being everything that I wasn't and for seemingly getting everything I ever wanted while I stood in the background, cheering her on. Looking back, I can see that a lot of anger and envy was bubbling under the surface leading up to that day when I hit her. It's a dynamic repeatedly portrayed in teen movies (Regina George and Gretchen Wieners, anyone?), and for a reason.

A few years later, after I'd moved away, we went back to visit our old friends. I can't remember the circumstance, but I ended up in a car with Shannen at one point, and there was an apology of sorts, which I accepted. It would have been foolish to harbour any resentment. These things happen when you're growing up and figuring things out. Still, I'll never forget the pain I felt in the aftermath of that friendship. (Shannen also revealed that the 'black eye' I had given her was the result of her mother's handiness with make-up!)

I've experienced the ending of friendships a few times in

my life. Sometimes, I've been the ender; sometimes, I've been the endee. Once, I ended a friendship with someone and, as a result, she ended my friendship with someone else. It's painful and I think, for the most part, it's unique to women. Our friendships are intense and loving. We care for each other so deeply and share so much, that when it's over there are not only the hurt feelings but also the pain of the absence.

Invisible me

People always ask me the same question about my time in high school in America: 'Is it like it is on TV?' My answer is, generally, yes. In many ways, it is. There are the cheerleaders and the jocks at the top of the food chain. They hang out together, with different guys taking turns to be the 'big man on campus', depending on what sport is in season. Basketball was important, but football was number one, really. In my school, the girls who excelled at sport were also popular and hung out with the 'cool kids'. What year you were in was not a factor, as classes in high schools in America are mixed in age. There are certain courses you need to take during your four years at high school, but in many cases it doesn't matter when you take them. So, you might decide you are going to take Communications in your freshman (first) year of high school, but someone else might decide to take it in their senior (last) year. As a result of these mixed classes, and mixed after-school activities, where students were grouped based on ability rather than age, friendship groups were mixed in age, too.

Much like the jocks and the cheerleaders, people tended to hang around together based on which after-school activities they did – being in the marching band or the choir, for example – though some people managed to belong to several groups. The coolest people were virtually card-carrying members of the 'in crowd' but also stars of the school choir. They were who I wanted to be. I wanted to be good at stuff, but still cool. Somehow, I managed to be fairly good at stuff, but invisible.

The legal driving age is sixteen in Chicago, so being in mixed-age social groups meant that, once you were in high school, you were independent. Groups of pals could drive themselves around – to the cinema, to parties, to each other's house. And yes, to football games, basketball games and pep rallies, all of which really were a big deal. Everyone went to them. (Except the group who would be labelled 'stoners' in a teen movie. They did their own thing and always absolutely terrified me.)

Homecoming week was a big deal every year, with alumni of the school returning to show everyone how brilliantly they were doing. In honour of this, there was a week of activities designed to celebrate the school spirit, from days themed around what we wore to school to a parade through the town with elaborate floats built by each year group. It all culminated in a big football game on Friday night, at which the homecoming court (a prince and princess from each year and an overall king and queen) was literally paraded around the stadium to rapturous applause. Afterwards there was a dance, at which attendees had to wear formal dress.

I still think it's utter bollocks that you have to have a date to go to a school dance. Why put that pressure on young people when they're at their least confident?

I loved every bit of homecoming week and was always heavily involved in the building of the float and any other element of it I could volunteer for. However, when it was time for the dance on the Saturday night, I stayed at home. Tickets could be bought only in pairs, and I never had anyone to go with. It sounds tragic, because it is! I still think it's utter bollocks that you have to have a date to go to a school dance. You don't need a date for any activity in adult life any more, so why put that pressure on young people when they're at their least confident?

Anyway, yes, American high school *is* like it is on TV. And yes, if you're an outsider, it can be almost unbearable. Which brings me back to the miserable life I found myself living after I 'broke up' with Shannen Walsh.

I had spent so many years joined at the hip to Shannen that I didn't really know who I was when our friendship ended. With Shannen, I was the smart one. The quieter one. The one who followed. My identity had been so linked to hers that I found myself bewildered. I had eaten lunch at school with her. I had passed her notes. I had hung out with her after school and at the weekend. All of that was gone. I wasn't sure how to go about my life.

I wasn't completely on my own; I still had acquaintances to chat to in class and groups to hang on the periphery of during lunch. But when I got home I was alone. I think it was around this time that I really fell in love with TV. Without a companion, I found myself watching it for hours (or as many hours as my parents would let me). The American daytime talk show was having a moment so, if I was lucky and my mom wasn't home after school, I would plonk my arse down on the couch and bunker in for hours of Ricki Lake, Sally Jessy Raphael, Jerry Springer and, at a push, Geraldo Rivera. My icon was Oprah, but her show was on while I was at school so I only got to watch it if there happened to be a repeat. I would keep the volume low so that I would hear my mother's car pull into the driveway. As soon as I heard the sound of the motor, I would switch the TV off and make a mad dash for my room, hoping I hadn't left behind any evidence of whatever I had been eating. These days, my favourite television features real people, which makes sense when I think back to those hours spent fantasizing about someday having my own talk show.

Once I was in my bedroom, I turned to other distractions. I devoured Danielle Steel novels, though each book had essentially the same plot. And the angry and unhappy songs of Fiona Apple and Alanis Morissette suited my mood and I listened to *Tidal* and *Jagged Little Pill* hundreds, if not thousands, of times.

My real escape at that time, however, was make-up. I wanted to be pretty and glamorous, and make-up seemed like the way to do it. I didn't really have any money, apart from the small sums I managed to pick up from babysitting. What was a girl who couldn't afford make-up to do? Well, I'm not proud of it, but I stole it. Lots of it. Nothing expensive, but enough that I could achieve almost any look I wanted. I think I felt entitled to it. I'd been living with my parents for about five years, and things had been financially tight for the duration. Having come from a, frankly, spoiled life I had found it really difficult to adjust. In Ireland, not only had Dee enjoyed buying me nice things and making me look pretty but, as I was the first-born grandchild on both sides, treats and gorgeous clothes were plentiful. With Ruaidhrí and Ger, there was no spoiling. They simply couldn't afford it. Being a moody adolescent, I concluded that

> *I wanted to be pretty and glamorous, and make-up seemed like the way to do it. What was a girl who couldn't afford make-up to do? Well, I'm not proud of it, but I stole it. Lots of it.*

I was hard done by. *Why does everyone else get to have nice things? Why am I the badly dressed girl at school? Why can't I be cool?* I wasn't able – or didn't have the balls – to steal clothes. In any case, due to my girth, I couldn't shop in trendy places like other girls of my age. On the other hand, make-up went on my face easily. So make-up became the hot-ticket item.

Once I had assembled my collection I would sit in front of my mirror and turn myself into someone else. I would picture someone in my head – from women I'd seen in sexy magazines while sneaking a peak at a friend's house to actresses I'd seen at the Oscars ceremony on TV – and try to copy their look. These were the most glamorous women I could think of, which says a lot about what I was exposed to as a thirteen-year-old growing up in America's Midwest. I did this for months, for hours and hours every weekend. These days, when people ask me how I acquired my make-up skills, I say, 'I didn't have any friends for six months when I was a teenager.' They laugh, but it's the truth.

To this day, make-up is a great comfort. It's not that I'm afraid to be seen bare-faced; I am quite happy to leave the house without it. Rather it's the process of applying make-up that I really enjoy. I find it relaxing, almost meditative. I guess it was a form of mindfulness before I knew what mindfulness was. In a world where we are rarely focused on just one thing at a time, make-up forces you to concentrate on the task in hand.

Aside from enjoying the artistry of doing my face, I also associated looking good and being pretty with my value as a person – not unusual for a girl of my age, but still kind of sad. I knew I was smart. I knew I could sing well and act reasonably well. I was 'talented'. But none of that meant anything if I wasn't pretty. And, anyway, I didn't have any friends, so what good was being clever and talented doing me?

Things I know at 33 that I wish I'd known at 18
(For my sister Aoife)

- The people who are the coolest in school are rarely the coolest ten years on.
- You are way, way more attractive than you think.
- Just because he likes you doesn't necessarily mean you like him.
- Sexy time isn't just about him enjoying himself; you should be having a good time, too.
- Talking about people behind their backs never, *ever* ends well.
- If the people around you don't enjoy the stuff you enjoy, find other people who do.
- Ignore the inner voice that says, 'You can't'; chances are, you can and, even if you can't, you'll learn something from trying.
- Unless you dedicate your entire life to looking good, you will never look as good as professionally good-looking people, because they have dedicated their entire life to looking that way. Have fun instead.
- There will always be someone with something nasty to say, but you're better off ignoring them.
- If someone you don't like doesn't like you, there's no reason to care.
- Not everyone is going to like you, and that's okay.
- There is definitely someone out there right this very minute who fancies you. I promise.
- Some people are just jerks.

Finding God (yes, really)

One night I remember sitting in my bedroom and hearing my next-door neighbour and some friends leaving to go out for the night. I went to the window and looked out between the curtains, hoping they might see me and ask me to go with them but knowing deep down they never would.

I felt lost and lonely. Things at home weren't great at the time, and I felt disconnected from everyone and everything. All the other kids at school seemed to be having the time of their lives. The high-school year had just started, and it was a flurry of football games and social events, and I had no one to invite me to them and no one to go with.

My neighbour's name was Andrea Smith. She was everything I was not and everything I wished I was. She was thin and good at sports. She lived in a beautiful house with a glamorous mom. She had the best clothes, the best hair, the best nail polish. She was funny and smart, and everyone liked her because she was also nice. She was the popular girl who said hi to you in the halls. She was one year above me in school, and when she got to high school she discovered she could sing as well and got into the show choir. Not the girls' one which you were lucky to get into when you were a freshman but the really good one that even people who thought show choir was lame quietly respected. There were only about twenty students in it, and they all seemed sophisticated and grown up. Places were hotly contested in annual auditions and, every once in a while, by fluke, someone who wasn't cool or popular would get in and – hey presto – become cool and popular. Does it sound like something from *Glee* or *Pitch Perfect*? That's because it *was* like something from *Glee* or *Pitch Perfect*.

Anyway, Andrea was always nice to me. Occasionally, all the neighbourhood kids would come together for a game of basketball, or an ultra-tough sport we called rugby but which was really just an excuse for us to run around and wrestle each other to the ground. When Andrea got into singing, our relationship changed. She could play the piano and, sometimes, if she was bored she'd call me and I'd go next door, where she'd play show tunes and we'd sing together. I still feel a real warmth remembering those times. I loved the singing itself, and it was unbelievably gratifying to feel visible for a moment to someone who was cool and popular. We developed a sort of friendship through this time spent together. Since it was only a home-time friendship – at school, we were still very much separate – when she invited me to go to church with her, I said yes.

Andrea's family were Christian, the kind of Christian which meant Andrea's younger brother wasn't allowed to read Harry Potter because it was about . . . 'witchcraft!' Their church had a youth group which met every week, mostly made up of kids from my high school but also some others in the surrounding area. Well, I loved it. All the kids who went shared the kind of confidence Andrea had. They were all nice, kind and welcoming. The sort of welcoming that comes from being raised in a house where being an evangelist is part of your upbringing. As I got to know Christians I realized they had a sense of obligation about showing warmth and hospitality both to those who had found Jesus and those who might yet do so.

Aside from that, youth group was fun! There were organized activities and everything was run by a youth minister employed by the church whose sole responsibility was to lead young people in their Christianity. Every youth minister I ever met was a cool, good-looking guy in his twenties with a beautiful wife. Really, I suppose, they were exactly what the young people were supposed to aspire to be. They certainly seemed to be living the dream to me at the time.

After going to youth group with Andrea a couple of times I was invited to go away with the group for a weekend. It was some sort of Christian teen convention, and I, happy to be included in anything, begged my parents for permission to go. For the first time in ages, I felt I fitted in. People seemed excited that I was there, and I really enjoyed myself over the weekend, which was one part disco, one part concert, one part evangelism. At the end, I stood in a crowd of hundreds of teenagers while a minister stood on the stage talking about how Jesus wanted everyone to love him and to accept him into their heart. The man asked anyone who wanted to come forward to accept Jesus to do so, and I found myself doing it. I was scared, but all I wanted was to feel secure and loved, so who was I to turn it down?

The man asked anyone who wanted to come forward to accept Jesus to do so, and I found myself doing it.

The people from the youth group were thrilled. People kept talking about how I'd feel different now and how my life was about to change. I felt a little scared, if I'm honest. What had I got myself into? Still, I did what they told me to do, and prayed and strained to feel this incredible feeling everyone had promised I would feel. Most of all, I waited to turn into a happy, confident teenager like the others in the youth group.

When I returned to school the following week I had a new gang of friends. People were looking out for me, calling me to sit with them at lunch, inviting me to hang out after school and at the weekend. This went beyond the people who'd been away on the weekend with me: word had spread through the wide network of Christians in my town, and it was obvious that parents had instructed their children to support me in my new journey. From then on, I went to church every Sunday and youth group every week. I started singing at church and rehearsing with my friends a couple of times a week.

I loved my new life. I loved being included and having new friends. I had a social life again, and I even got my first boyfriend, even if it was just a bit of hand-holding and we only lasted a couple of weeks. The thing is, though, as much as I wanted to have faith, I didn't. I had questions. I never really felt anything when I prayed. The people at church were encouraging me to be baptized, but I kept making excuses. I just couldn't seem to believe.

About a year into my voyage with born-again Christianity, my parents announced that we were moving to England. At this stage, we were a family of six – I had two little sisters, Úna and Aoife. My parents wanted to move closer to Ireland to be nearer to their ageing parents and to make sure that we had the option of going to college. In America, parents have to save from the moment their children are born in order to be able to afford third-level education, and my parents were not in a position to fund an American college education for four children. The move was for my own good but I didn't see it like that. I was just about to turn sixteen! I was about to

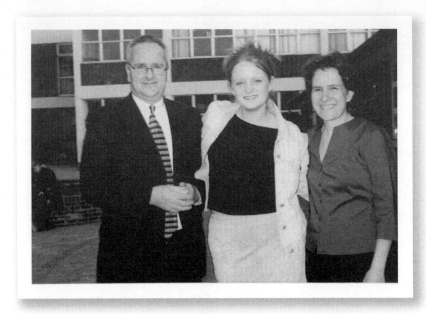

With my dad and mom, Ruaidhrí and Ger McSharry, at my school graduation, Dublin, 2001.

start driving! And I had only just got my social life back! I was angry and indignant, and felt these things deeply. What I admitted only to myself was that I was also kind of relieved. I didn't want to leave the community aspect of church behind – I had found it incredibly heartening – but I didn't know how long I could carry on the charade. Even now, I feel guilty about it.

My church friends threw a surprise going-away party for me. They were all really lovely. They told me to 'find a church'. That should be my first priority. There was a part of me that genuinely thought I might do it, too. Maybe I'd get there? Maybe I'd find faith for real?

It probably won't come as a surprise that I didn't make finding a church my first priority when we got to England. I did go to a Christian church in Dublin a couple of times when we moved back to Ireland a year later, but by then I knew that it just wasn't going to happen for me. As much as I envied the lives of those who had faith and belonged to warm Christian communities, it just wasn't me.

As much as I envied the lives of those who had faith and belonged to warm Christian communities, it just wasn't me.

Realistically, I was never going to be able to get onboard with many elements of that type of religion. I love gay people and see them as my equals. I am pro-choice. I am a feminist. This doesn't mean that I don't feel a real warmth towards people who have faith and live a happy, loving life within that. There are many great people who are religious but do not feel the need to stand in judgement of others. My great-aunt Mary, for example, was a nun. She must have had certain beliefs that would not be consistent with mine, but she never felt the need to force them on me. In her family circle children were born in loving relationships but outside marriage and she accepted and loved them without reserve. She was a generous, kind and joyful person.

At breakfast on what turned out to be the last day of Mary's life she said she felt a bit funny and was going to go for a lie-down. One of the other sisters walked her up the stairs. On the way, Mary turned to her and said, 'Do you know, I feel I'll be with Sister Agnes soon.' Sister Agnes was a member of the order who had died a few months earlier. Great-aunt Mary then got into her bed, fell asleep and never woke up. I don't know about you, but I find much to envy about that. Imagine sensing that your time is coming and feeling no fear? That is a truly special thing.

2
Sex

When will I be loved (or at least kissed)?

I'm not sure exactly when I became aware of sex, but I know that by the time I was seven I knew it was something that men and women did together when they really, really liked each other. I had started drawing crude pictures of men and women together in my diary, and my mother, somewhat amused, had taken me to task about it. What did I know about sex?

Sex education was thoroughly covered in health class in my American high school, and what I didn't learn there I began to glean from the filthy book a classmate had stolen from her mother's bedroom and took great pleasure in reading aloud from on the school bus and at lunchtime.

I managed to procure a dirty book of my own from the house of a family I babysat for (sorry, guys). The book was *Men in Love* by the American author Nancy Friday. It was, in theory, an analysis of men's sexual fantasies. In reality, it was an education in all the very different ways people had sex and all the different things men were into. It was probably not the best way for a thirteen-year-old to learn about such matters, but it was all I had at the time, and I devoured it. And when I say 'devoured' I mean that I read it from cover to cover several times (skipping the boring psychological talk), deciding which bits were my favourites and then going back to those favourite bits again and again over the course of a few years.

It's a pity that the book was filled with men's sexual fantasies, because I was struggling to believe that any boy or man

> **On some level I knew I was pretty, but my stupid, fat body was certainly not good enough to be fancied.**

would ever fancy me. On some level I knew I was pretty, but my stupid, fat body was certainly not good enough to be fancied. No boy had ever expressed any interest in me, and it seemed that boyfriends and crushes were the territory of my thinner, better-dressed friends. Like most girls that age, I wanted things to be different and puzzled over what I could do to make boys like me. Could there possibly be a way to compensate for my gross body? Would there ever be a day someone might fancy me?

I found it hard to believe the answer to either of those questions could ever be 'yes'. Just in case you are reading this and feeling this way about yourself, I want to take a moment here to tell you that you are wrong. I was wrong, too. I'm not saying there were hundreds of guys who fancied me, but there were some. They've come out of the woodwork over the years to say sheepishly, 'I really fancied you in school.' I always think, *'Jesus, why couldn't you have told me?'* Because it would have made a huge difference to how I felt about myself. I wish it hadn't been that way, and that my self-worth hadn't been so reliant on the way I thought boys saw me, but it was. It was very important to me. So, if it's important to you, please know that there is almost certainly someone, right now, who fancies you. You might not fancy them but, someday, someone who you fancy will also fancy you, and it will be wonderful. The very worst things you think about yourself are almost certainly inaccurate. Be kind to yourself. Your day will come. (In fact, some of the people you wish you could be right now might well be having the best time of their lives and later it will all be downhill for them. Your best days are still ahead of you.)

But, anyway, back to sex.

Because I had very little self-esteem, when I thought about sex I thought about it being the ultimate vote of confidence a woman could receive from a man. Surely if someone was willing to have sex with me, then I was okay? Right? I was desperate for any kind of indication that I wasn't a complete turn-off and, unfortunately, I wasn't getting it.

I didn't experience any form of physical affection until I was nearly sixteen, not long after we moved to England. I was attending the house party of someone I didn't really know with my friend Karen, and we had managed to procure a bottle of vermouth, believing it to be the sophisticate's drink of choice. I walked into the party wearing a fur-trimmed black cardigan, seventy-five butterfly hair ornaments and enough glitter hairspray to asphyxiate a small nation. It seemed like it was going to be just another night of basking in my friend's confidence and popularity when, out of nowhere, a boy was talking to me. Yes, he was just acting as a good wingman for the guy who was going after Karen, but still, he was paying me attention! The four of us sat on the stairs chatting, but not for long. Karen and Guy Number One started wearing the faces off each other. I was very afraid because I knew what was going to happen, and I wasn't sure if I was ready. And then I was doing it. It was happening. His tongue was in my mouth and I wasn't sure if I liked it but WHO THE HELL CARED? SOMEONE'S TONGUE WAS IN MY MOUTH!

His tongue was in my mouth and I wasn't sure if I liked it but WHO THE HELL CARED? SOMEONE'S TONGUE WAS IN MY MOUTH!

The romance was interrupted briefly when he foolishly attempted to touch my hair. I brushed his hand away, genuinely afraid it might get stuck in the glittery jungle of butterflies. 'It's crispy with glitter,' I said.

'It is,' he replied.

After a period of kissing on the stairs, it was time for us to go home. We were fifteen, after all, and had parents to answer to. All at once, things changed. Karen's guy was still charming away, but my one wasn't even looking at me any more. In fact, he seemed aggrieved when his friend suggested that a group of us walk home together. I wasn't put off, though. It was probably just that he wasn't into public displays of affection. He probably just felt uncomfortable in front of his mates. I walked home with the group of guys and Karen, feeling positively sparkling. I had been kissed! I was okay! This was the start of the rest of my life! He grunted goodbye when we arrived at my house, and I crept into the room I shared with my sister, struggling to contain squeals of excitement. It was happening at last. Everything had changed.

The next day I positively bounded out of my bed and down the stairs to ring Karen for the rehash. She'd been on the phone already. Apparently, people were talking. My guy had a girlfriend. I said the kind of things I'd heard people say on TV, about how unfair it was on her and that I felt guilty. (I did not feel guilty at all; in fact, I was somewhat thrilled by the prospect of being 'the other woman'.) I wondered if he would break up with his girlfriend, although they'd been together for several months, an eternity in my fifteen-year-old mind.

The sparkle had dulled somewhat, but I felt sure things would work out for the best. It probably won't surprise you to hear they didn't. I never heard from him again.

When I turned sixteen later that year, I remember my aunt saying to me, 'Sweet sixteen and never been kissed! I doubt that's true!' I savoured the knowledge that she was right. Even if that guy had turned out to be a bit of a jerk, at least I wasn't turning sixteen like some sort of weirdo, without ever having kissed someone.

My perspective didn't change much between my sixteenth birthday and the night I lost my virginity when I was seventeen. The guy was a friend of a friend. I barely knew him. I did it because he wanted to and because I wanted to get it out of the way. It was another thing to add to the list of things I used to attempt to reassure myself that I was normal and not the monster I felt like most of the time. The sex was barely functional; my body was not prepared to let this happen in the laissez-faire manner my heart was. Still, I walked home the next day with a pep in my step. Someone had had sex with me. I wasn't revolting, after all.

The dickhead years

Once I became sexually active, a pattern developed. On a night out, or at a party, a guy would show interest in me. I would be thrilled and, without considering for a moment whether or not I was interested in him, I would go along with whatever it was he wanted to do. Each and every time, I would convince myself that this time would be different, that this was definitely going to be the beautiful relationship I longed for – and each and every time, I would be disappointed. Frequently, the guys would assist me in my fantasy by telling me what I wanted to hear – that I was special, beautiful, that they cared about me, etcetera – but ninety-nine per cent of the time, the dream was entirely my own.

It's really sad for me to look back on these times and on the way I felt about myself. I doubt very much that I was alone or was unique in my way of thinking. I'd really like to think that, if I can get to the bottom of what was behind it for me, I might be able to help the young women I meet.

So what was it that made me feel that I was disgusting? What was it that had me convinced that no one would ever fancy me? And why was I basing my entire self-worth on whether or not guys found me attractive?

The first question is easy to answer. I felt I was disgusting because that's what the world was telling me and I believed it. The way society feels about fat women is very clear. Fat women are a joke (Fat Monica in *Friends*). Fat women are odious (Melissa McCarthy's character in *Bridesmaids*). Fat women are unlovable (*Shallow Hal* – the plot revolves around the eponymous Hal's struggle to come to terms with a woman's fatness because she has such a gosh-darned sweet personality; the main character is played by a far from skinny Jack Black whose fatness is ignored).

Which brings me to question two. Every film, book and television show I had ever seen had sent me the clear message that the fat girl never gets the guy. In fact, the fat girls are invisible to guys. Except when they're the butt of the joke. That message had been driven home for me in real life, too, by the guys who shouted at me at the bus stop, who said I smelled, who called me disgusting, who scrawled FAT GIRL in giant black permanent-marker letters on my school bag. Oh, I knew my place.

Every film, book and television show I had ever seen had sent me the clear message that the fat girl never gets the guy.

As for basing my self-worth on whether or not boys fancied me – well, I think that's an issue lots of young women face. Beauty is seen as the most desirable characteristic they can have, and it's measured in attention. It didn't matter if I was the smartest, or the best singer, or the most articulate in my class. In fact, those things seemed to intimidate some of my male classmates. 'Shut up, Louise, no one wants to hear what you have to say,' was what one of them said to me one day in sixth year back in Dublin when I was taking part in an English class. I enjoyed English. I enjoyed participating. But even that wasn't okay in the eyes of this guy. And he was one of the intelligent ones. Everything I was and did seemed to be the wrong thing. How could I possibly feel good about myself? It was no wonder I craved any form of approval from the opposite sex, even if what

I viewed as approval was in fact guys using me whenever it suited them.

It wasn't until I was in my twenties that things changed. And it wasn't finding a genuinely loving and respectful relationship that did it, although that was pretty good. Instead, it was a surprising conversation at a time when the last thing I was expecting was a profound shift in the way I thought about men.

It all went back to a 'relationship' I had had during my fleeting stay in UCD. I say 'relationship' tentatively because, while it met some of the criteria of what you'd recognize as a relationship (i.e. I obsessed about him and we had sex reasonably regularly over the space of six months), it wasn't the kind of relationship I needed at the time.

One day I turned on my phone to find seventeen missed calls from a guy who was harassing me. I was telling a friend all about it, probably loving the drama. A guy interjected in what seemed like a very manly fashion, to ask if I'd like him to tell the harasser to back off. To an attention-starved eighteen-year-old, this seemed like the ultimate act of chivalry. Was he tall, dark and handsome? Well, he was tall and dark. Later that night in the student bar he was relentless in his pursuit, even though I was there with someone else. I *know*! Two guys interested in me at the same time. I could hardly believe my luck.

The someone else I was with had one too many and had to go home. I missed my last bus. One thing led to another with my would-be rescuer. I was initially uncertain but the next day my brain kicked into its usual fantasy mode and I decided I fancied him. This time, it seemed like he might fancy me as well.

A few days later I was at a party when he pulled me to one side for a chat. I had been here before. This time, the story was that he still had feelings for his ex. I was great and all, but he wasn't interested. By this stage, I was good at remaining dignified in rejection and managed to hold it together until I got to the toilets for the traditional cry. Determined not to let him see I was bothered, I returned to the party and made it look like I was having the time of my life. By the end of the night, he was back by my side, and on the journey to the after-party he tried to hold my hand. I briefly thought I had the upper hand and said, 'I thought you weren't interested?' He laughed. I went home with him again that night.

That pattern carried on for a good six months. He wasn't interested, but he was interested. He didn't want anything like a relationship with me, but he wanted me to come home with him at the end of the night when he felt like it. Sometimes, he feigned genuine interest in me; other times, he was much more transparent. I wish I could say I ended it, but I didn't, though my friends begged me to. As one of them said at the time, he was 'one charming motherfucker'.

It did end, however. I can't remember the specifics, but I do remember one dramatic moment at a house party when the floodlights in the back garden came on, illuminating a couple locked in a passionate embrace – 'my' charming man with a girl I considered a friend.

At a Christmas party about five years later I got chatting to a guy who had been in college with me. We were not particularly close but we had known each other for a long time. Whatever we were talking about he turned to me and said, 'Louise, I swear to God, if I ever see you letting a guy treat you the way Dweebus did in college, I'll kick your ass. That was disgraceful.' I was shocked, and stuttered something in reply, but I also felt a strange warmth spread through me as the conversation returned to normal. *Someone had noticed!*

Someone had noticed that what that guy had done wasn't right. What he had done had *not* been right. I had not been right to allow it to continue. I deserved better.

I deserved better.

It was a life-changing moment for me. It's sad that it took the words of a relative stranger to get me there, but at least I got there in the end. From then on, I never had relations with anyone I didn't fancy and have feelings for . . . And if you believe that, you'd believe anything!

However, I did start to consider my needs and put myself in fewer and fewer dangerous, hurtful situations. It was only then that I realized I had never really considered what I wanted in bed. I had spent my entire life thinking about what I could do to please whoever I was with in order to make them like me, and never really thought about what worked for me. In fact, I don't even think I had really considered whether or not I even fancied whoever it was in the first place. My entire focus had been on what they thought of me, whether they liked me, whether they were being pleased by me. My happiness and desires were not even a factor. How tragic is that?

I think a lot about the way women – particularly, young women – think about sex. I wonder if, like me, their own satisfaction is frequently an afterthought, and if there are lots of women who go through their entire lives never really asking for what they want. I once lived with two women, neither of whom had ever had an orgasm. They were in their twenties. They had had boyfriends, and they had never had an orgasm. Find me a man in his twenties who has had a girlfriend and has never had an orgasm! You won't, because they don't exist. Not only do women feel it is their responsibility to provide an orgasm, men demand them.

Men know what works for them because it is considered

normal for them to explore their sexuality as they grow up. The opposite is true for women. Happily, this is changing, as more and more women claim their space in the discussion of sexuality. These days, many women are speaking freely about their experiences and demanding more and more out of their encounters. This delights me.

I think there are still lots of young women who feel as if the primary aim of a heterosexual encounter is to please their mate, and I can only imagine that the ubiquity of porn is making that even worse. In my day, women's challenge was to master the blow job. *More!* magazine and *Basic Instinct* were the handiest sources of guidance on sexual skills. Now, in the era of the internet, boys and girls are seeing every type of sexual encounter imaginable (and some hardly imaginable), and things that were once taboo are now mundane. I believe it means that young men have unrealistic expectations when it comes to sex, and young women are pushing themselves to satisfy crazier and crazier demands. I dread to think what I might have done in my desperation to please when I was a teenager, and what lasting impact some of that could have had on me.

When given the opportunity to speak to young women I find myself desperately telling them that they are the prize.

When given the opportunity to speak to young women – and it's usually my cousins (apologies, cousins . . . and extra apologies, because this always seems to happen when I've had a few gins) – I find myself desperately telling them that they are the prize. I tell them they are precious, and that if they are wanted by boys they have the power to dictate how the encounter goes. They can and should ask for what they want, and they should never push themselves beyond what they're comfortable with, because the boys are lucky to be with them in the first place.

I want young women to feel valuable and special. I want them to know that teenage boys are often idiots, that they should place their own happiness before anything else and that if they do that they will have fulfilling relationships. I don't want them to make the same mistakes I did. I want them to feel important, because they are.

Yes, all women

I was six, I remember, the first time a man made me feel uncomfortable with his inappropriate behaviour. I was sitting in the car with Andrew when an adult man walked by and mimed cunnilingus at me through the window. I felt frightened, but I wasn't sure why. When Dee returned to the car I asked her what the gesture he had made meant. I saw anger flash across her face and then she explained that the man was just being yucky.

It was a quick thing, but the feeling of violation has stayed with me my entire life. Any time a man has acted inappropriately towards me in a similar fashion, that man's face has flashed up in my mind's eye. There was the time I was sixteen and on my way to my Irish-dancing class and a man at least forty years my senior sat beside me in a deserted train carriage, put his hand on my knee and asked me if I had a boyfriend.

Three years later, on a jam-packed DART, a drunken man shouted that he 'knew who I was', he 'knew what I'd done'. He then sat on my lap, licked my face and groped my breasts. No one said anything, including the man who was sitting right beside me and had been chatting to me before the arrival of the drunkard. '*I DON'T KNOW YOU!*' I shouted. '*YOU CAN'T DO THIS TO ME!*' Eventually, I managed to use the momentum of the train stopping to shove him off me. He stumbled off the DART at the next stop. I sat there, red-faced and seething. I turned to the man beside me and said,

'Really?! You did nothing?' He couldn't even meet my gaze.

A couple of years ago I went to the cinema on my own (something I really enjoy doing, by the way; don't fear it, it's great, usually). I went to see *The Fault in Our Stars* on a weekday afternoon. The cinema was almost empty. About an hour into the film a man got up from his seat a few rows in front of me and came to sit right beside me. From time to time he moved his knee towards mine, rubbing it against me, while I turned as far away from him as I could. I was frozen in panic. I wanted to run away but, for some reason, I was worried about offending him. What if he had a disability? What if he didn't really know what he was doing? I searched my mind for a reasonable explanation of this situation, which had made me so deeply uncomfortable, trying to believe it wasn't just that he was an absolute creep. But he probably *was* just a creep.

I was covering for Ryan Tubridy that week on 2fm, so I mentioned my experience on air. Texts flew in. Some people had had similar experiences, felt the same way and sympathized with me. Others said I had overreacted. 'You wouldn't have been bothered if yer man was good-looking,' one person said. That made me angry. How could this person miss the point so completely? First of all, I hadn't even really seen the man's face in the darkness of the cinema, so his appearance was irrelevant. Second, and more importantly, even if he had been the most attractive man in the world, he was a stranger who took it upon himself to invade my personal space and touch me without my permission. It was just wrong and creepy.

The worst of these experiences took place when I was sixteen and living in England. I told my parents that I was going to stay at my friend Karen's house (I was; we just weren't planning to be there most of the night) and popped out the door on a Saturday afternoon. Once at Karen's, I got dolled up and we went out to meet two lads from our year in school. Really nice lads, it's important to say. We were going to a nightclub in a nearby town where they had a lenient door policy. Of course, being sixteen, we didn't realize that nightclubs don't open until 11 p.m., so we found ourselves with several hours to kill. We did what any sixteen-year-olds in the know would do: we went to the nearest supermarket, bought a bottle of Bacardi and a two-litre bottle of Coke and went to town (that we thought a two-litre bottle of Coke was enough mixer for an entire bottle of Bacardi shows how naïve we were). It didn't take long for the Bacardi to be gone.

I don't recall getting into the nightclub. Next thing I remember is buying a Bacardi Breezer, taking a sip and realizing things were not going to go well. I went to the toilet and threw up. Before I knew it, a security guard was carrying me out of the club. She plonked me down on the ground and left me there. Mobile phones were new at the time, and I didn't have one, so there was no way of contacting my friends. I just sat there, on my own, vomiting.

Though my memory of that night is blurry, some bits are very clear. I remember a man coming over and starting to talk to me. He asked me how old I was, and I told him. I asked him how old he was, and he told me he was twenty-five. After a couple of minutes he picked me up from the ground and brought me to a bench a little bit down the road. He continued to talk to me, telling me I was beautiful. I hadn't ever been told that by anyone who wasn't related to me. I knew it couldn't be true but still I basked in it. Every so often I vomited. This didn't seem to bother him, though, and he kissed me. It was only the second time I'd been kissed. I couldn't help but enjoy what felt to me like a vote of confidence in my worth as a woman.

My memory has more gaps about how long we spent on the bench and moving away from it. I remember coming to in a shop doorway around the corner. The man was sitting behind me with his legs wrapped around me, and the lads from school were standing over us, shouting at him. They pulled me up off the ground, and we hurried down the street. I panicked, now all too aware of how serious things could have been. I started babbling and crying; I was scared and aware that my friends were angry with me. We made our way home, and when I woke up at Karen's the next morning I was shaken. I couldn't say for sure what had happened. Possibly, nothing. I knew for sure, though, that if my friends hadn't come along, something terrible would have. In the cold light of day, the man seemed repulsive. What kind of twenty-five-year-old (if he even was twenty-five) was interested in a sixteen-year-old girl? What kind of man kissed a girl while she was vomiting? Karen didn't have any sympathy for me. She made it clear that I needed to shut up about it. So I did.

Of course, these are not the only experiences of this kind I've had. Like every woman, I have a litany of stories about when I felt violated, from a hand up my skirt in a crowd to a stranger grabbing my breasts on a dance floor. Every time, I've felt the same. Angry. Embarrassed. Shocked. And confused. Every single time, I've tried to come up with a reasonable explanation for unreasonable behaviour. Every time, I've racked my brain as to whether I was somehow to blame for the whole thing.

If you're a woman, I bet you know what I'm talking about. I bet you've felt the same. If you're a man, then you're probably thinking, I would never do that. I can't believe these things happen. But they do. To all women. In case you missed it, that's what caused the #yesallwomen hashtag to go viral on Twitter in 2014. It came in the aftermath of the murder of six people and the injury of fourteen others near the University of California, Santa Barbara. The killer, Elliot Rodger, committed suicide during the incident but left behind a video entitled 'Elliot Rodger's Retribution' in which he outlined his motivation for the killings. He wanted to punish women for rejecting him and to seek revenge against men who were more sexually successful than him. He hated women because he didn't get what he felt entitled to, and killed them as a result.

Such a high level of misogyny is disturbing to many men, because the hashtag #notallmen was launched. These men wanted people to know they weren't like Elliot Rodger. They wanted to clear their name. An anonymous female Twitter user started the #yesallwomen hashtag in response, and thousands of women all over the world tweeted about their experiences of misogyny and violence at the hands of men. In fact, 1.2 million tweets used the hashtag in the four days after it was created.

I am responsible for some of those 1.2 million tweets. I got involved because I know that not all men are misogynists. I know that not all men feel entitled to women's attention. I know that not all men view women as objects. However, all women have experienced misogyny. All women have been forced to pay attention to men they have no interest in. All

Not all men are misogynists. Not all men feel entitled to women's attention. Not all men view women as objects. However, all women have experienced misogyny.

women have been made to feel like objects. And all those men who are not responsible for such behaviour need to know that many of their counterparts are. They need to understand that when women talk about negative experiences at the hands of men it is not an attack on men in general but on behaviour that is extremely common.

The decent guys also need to accept that it is their responsibility to call out other men if they're being inappropriate with women. They must point out – to their mates, if needs be – that it's not cool to speak to and about women in a certain way and that it's not okay to be a creep.

I was at Oktoberfest in Dublin with my husband and some friends last autumn. We had reserved a table and were bunkered in for a good evening of strong beer and polka music when there was a little bit of aggro between him and a table of lads sitting behind us. I tried to intervene, because I'd seen them grab his arse out of the corner of my eye and thought it wasn't worth getting into a row over. As it turned out, I'd missed the main event. He'd seen one of the guys 'hilariously' pretending to put his finger up the bum of one of my female friends while she was standing up. My husband had told the guy to stop, and his response had been to wink at him, smile and run his finger under his nose, as if to smell it. The other lads at his table then laughed and started grabbing Gordon, possibly trying to defuse the situation.

When Gordon explained everything to me, I was furious on our friend's behalf, but I also felt uncomfortable. The thing is, when a man objectifies a woman like that he objectifies all the women around. I felt paranoid and that I had to stay sitting down. What had they said about me? What other gestures had they made while we weren't looking? Gordon tried to make me feel better by saying that he thought most of the lads at the table were sound, that there was just one jerk. It didn't work. Because none of those lads had intervened. None of them had told that one to leave it out. None of them had said, 'Come on, man, that's not cool.' Instead, they laughed. And their laughter sanctioned his behaviour.

Any reasonable person knows that that kind of carry-on is not cool. Whether you're talking about this Oktoberfest incident or the guy who sat on me on the train, the behaviour is not okay. The only way it's going to stop is if we are loud in our disapproval. That means women when it happens to us and men when they see it happening. If you ignore it when it happens, you're not a good guy just because you haven't done it yourself. It's not 'just a laugh'. It wouldn't be 'just a laugh' if it was your girlfriend, or your sister, or your mother. Or I should say *when* it is your girlfriend, *and* your sister, *and* your mother. Because these things have happened to them. No doubt about it.

3
Work

Falling in love with radio

I started working in radio when I was twenty. I had dropped out of college after failing to attend most of the lectures for the Arts degree I was meant to be doing. After being a bit of a teacher's pet in school I felt lost on the sprawling campus. I couldn't handle the feeling of anonymity in the giant lecture halls or the sense that it didn't really matter whether or not I turned up to class. I also wasn't all that interested in the degree itself. Having missed the Communications course I had wanted to do in DCU by five points, my choice came down to Arts in UCD or Audiovisual Communications in IT Tallaght. Based on the wonderful time my parents had had in UCD and some old-school South Dublin snobbery, I chose UCD. I don't want to say it was the wrong choice, because I suppose the path worked out for me, but if I had to make it again I think I would do it differently. I think I would have really enjoyed a few years of studying media, and I'd have a degree now.

While I didn't achieve much academically in UCD, I did have my first experience of radio in its student radio station. I signed up during Freshers' Week and was impressed by the guy who was acting as station manager that year. He was friendly and open and encouraged me to get involved, allowing me to present during a test broadcast ahead of the official fortnight of radio we were licensed to produce. For a couple of hours, I played my own CDs and talked about the songs, and I can honestly say I had never felt more at home anywhere. It sounds cheesy, because it is, but I truly felt I had found my calling.

I'm sure the station manager's mother was the only person listening that day, but she told her son that she thought I had 'a gift', and boy, did I latch on to that. There weren't many things I'd ever been naturally good at, aside from maybe English class in school, so the idea that radio presenting was something I possessed a natural talent for was exciting.

> *There weren't many things I'd ever been naturally good at, so the idea that radio presenting was something I possessed a natural talent for was exciting.*

Don't get me wrong: I'd been all right at lots of things during my school years, but I'd never been the best at anything. Now here was something I could excel at.

From then on, I was involved in any aspect of the station I could be, from writing and reading the news to presenting shows and organizing staff. This meant that when the shit hit the fan in terms of my academic career* I had another one in mind. I wasn't really sure how to get into radio professionally, though, and it was only when I volunteered to help at the Special Olympics World Games in the summer of 2003 that I made any progress. I was running the media desk in the National Basketball Arena and one of the girls I was working with was doing some work in Newstalk. I barely knew about the station's existence, and it certainly wasn't the music-radio

---

* By that, I mean I didn't bother to take my exams or tell my parents about this decision, leading to my dad finding out about this turn of events when he went to check my results while I was on holidays in Greece. I'm surprised he didn't manage to strangle me down the line.

job I had in mind, but she gave me the name of the station's editor and suggested they might let me do some work experience.

I sent him an email, and he replied with a very kind 'Thanks, but we get loads of these emails' response. Then I did something that was quite out of character for me but which I now view as one of the most important things I've ever done, though it was just sending an email. Rather than one of my usual meek 'Thanks so much for even deigning to email me' replies, I wrote back, 'Thank you, but I do hope you'll consider me. I promise that, if you take me on, you won't regret it.'

I'm not sure where the bolshiness came from, but I got a phone call the following week, and the week after that I started three weeks' work experience on David McWilliams' breakfast show.

When I say that I hadn't a notion when I walked in that first day, I *really* hadn't a notion. I didn't listen to the station. I had no idea who David McWilliams was. I didn't know anything about current affairs. However, I wasn't about to let them know that, and I bluffed my way through the morning, enjoying every moment. It was such a thrill to be involved in a live broadcast and, in a start-up station with limited resources, it was truly a case of all hands on deck, so the team wasn't shy about giving me work. When I left that day I had put together an item for the following day's show, about whether or not school uniforms should be banned.

For the first time in a long while, I felt like I was in the right place, and I spent the following weeks dashing home after work to study flashcards on the Oireachtas and brushing up on things I had heard mentioned in the station that morning. At the end of my three-week stint there was no mention of me finishing up, so I continued to arrive each morning at five thirty. When I went on a two-week holiday a few months later, they had to book another work-experience person to cover me, because I had made myself a part of the team: I had jobs that needed to be done and, if I was gone, I was missed. This is the way a lot of stories about radio careers begin, with people working for free and hanging around a station until they sort of slide into a job. It's not a perfect system, and it was certainly difficult to work a seven-hour shift in Newstalk before walking across town to do five hours' paid work in an office, but I wouldn't have given it up for the world. It was an incredible education and forced me to learn swiftly and thoroughly.

After six months, I started to be paid for research shifts, filling in for various members of staff when they were sick or on holidays. Soon I was working virtually full-time as a free-lance researcher within the station, and just over a year after I had started my work experience I was offered a full-time, permanent contract.

I spent four and a half years in Newstalk, working across several programmes of varying styles, with several present-ers ... of varying styles. I learned from each of them and have nothing but respect for all of them, particularly Orla Barry and George Hook, on whose shows I spent most of my time. They taught me to be conscientious and hard-working and that the easy way was often not the best way. Now, as a presenter, I feel I am definitely better for having worked my way up through the ranks. I know what it's like at each stage in the process of putting a show together, and I have an appreciation for each and every person in the team working on a programme.

Redundancy

Ever since I became a paragon of cancerous virtue, people have really enjoyed asking me what is the biggest challenge I've ever faced. The difficult childhood? Or the spot of bother with the life-threatening illness? I won't lie: I feel a real sense of cruel satisfaction when I surprise them by saying that it was neither of those things. Aside from the whole fatness thing, the most challenging thing I've encountered in my life is being made redundant.

Aside from the whole fatness thing, the most challenging thing I've encountered in my life is being made redundant.

After over four years in Newstalk I was ready for a change and thinking about exploring other opportunities when the station's former CEO happened to get in touch to tell me about a new project he was working on. He was starting a radio station for young people in the west of Ireland and wanted to meet for a chat. A few chats later, I had signed up to move to Galway and be involved in the creation of iRadio. I was really excited to move there. I had just ended a serious relationship, so the idea of a fresh start was appealing. And the prospect of being involved in a radio project from the ground up was incredibly exciting.

At the time I joined the team it consisted only of the station's owners and two employees. I spent the following months working to devise the news and speech content of the station, assisting in programme creation and travelling the country to meet potential staff. During this time I was also involved in the company's application to win another radio licence to broadcast to the north-east of Ireland, and I presented part of the company's application at the Broadcasting Authority of Ireland's oral hearing. It was heady stuff. I was eating, sleeping and breathing iRadio, and I loved it.

During this time, we were trying out different people for presenting roles on the station. We had done an open talent search and were meeting with lots of people who had personality but no real experience. I recorded mock programmes with each of them to see what they would be like in a double-header situation. These recordings led to me being asked to leave the management role I was in and to become the presenter of the breakfast show.

It was a difficult decision. I wanted to be in a management role in radio, but I had always wanted to be a presenter along the way. Should I stay where I was, in a relatively secure position, and skip the presenting portion of my career? Or should I take the opportunity to present?

I chose the presenting role. I wasn't a hundred per cent confident that it was the right decision, but I couldn't be sure I wouldn't regret it if I didn't give it a go.

The new station performed in terms of gaining listeners; the owners even launched the second station for the north-east. But, due to the economic crash, it struggled commercially. Advertising revenue had plummeted in every station in Ireland, and we were no different. In March 2010 staff were called into a meeting to be told that things were going to change. The two stations were going to be merged somewhat, with the Galway studios closed and broadcasting continuing solely from Athlone. There were going to be twelve redundancies.

I immediately put on my 'supportive leader' head and volunteered to be the staff representative who would ensure proper communication throughout the thirty-day redundancy process. I felt it was my responsibility, since I had been involved in hiring so many of the people in the station. Given my history with the company, I never thought for one second that I would be one of the people to be let go. I was wrong.

On the day the redundancies were announced, we were all called to individual meetings with one of the co-founders of the company and an external HR rep who was there to assist in the process. The meetings took place in a cold, sterile room in a hotel, and the entire thing felt utterly clinical. Upon sitting down, we were read a list of criteria, based on which we could earn points. Those who did not have sufficient points were being let go. The points criteria were a source of much debate at the time. You could get points for having experience in news and current affairs, for example, something lots of staff had. However, you could also get points for being a stand-up comedian or a part-time DJ, as those activities were seen to promote the company. I was not a stand-up comedian, and I did not DJ at night-time (my 5 a.m. starts were not conducive to such activities). So, I did not have sufficient points. I couldn't believe it, and I didn't even attempt to hide my feelings about it. 'After all this,' I said, 'after everything, it comes down to this BULLSHIT?' They say you shouldn't take these things personally, but this felt very, very personal.

They say you shouldn't take these things personally, but this felt very, very personal.

I think they would have preferred if I had just gone then, but I wanted to do the show another time, and so did my co-presenter, Conor Lynch, whose role was being restructured and who would no longer be doing the show. We were forbidden to mention that things were changing, so as we finished up the show for the last time, after two and a half years of going to work with our listeners, we couldn't say goodbye. Instead, we said a heartfelt 'Thanks a million for listening, it really means a lot,' and went on our way. I do not understand why we were not allowed to say it was our last show. Maybe it was feared we would bad-mouth the station, but I would never have done that. I cared too much about the colleagues I was leaving behind.

Looking back at emails from that time, I'm surprised at how positive I seem. I guess, initially, I thought I was going to be fine. I sent my demo out to radio stations in Dublin and I was happy to be moving back. I had been seeing a guy for a year and was head over heels in love. Gordon worked in RTÉ, so our relationship had been restricted to weekends. We were sick of travelling back and forth and ready to live in the same city. I got some work with 2fm relatively fast, doing my first show on the station in August. It was only the occasional slot filling in for people who were off or on holidays.

My confidence had taken a huge hit and, when I moved back to Dublin, I fell into a major rut. I moved into a house with two friends, which should have been great, but I felt like I had nothing to say to them, as I spent more and more time in bed on my laptop and less and less time out in the real world. I applied for lots of jobs, rarely getting a response and, frankly, giving out an air of unattractive desperation when I did get an interview. I found it difficult to find any

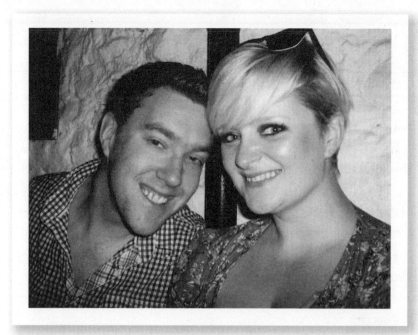

Gordon and me, 2010.

motivation to do anything at all and found myself closing my bedroom door each evening when my friends got home from work, too ashamed to reveal that I was still in my pyjamas, having barely moved since they had left that morning.

This went on for a few months, until I decided that something had to change. For me, there is nothing better than opening up about something that's bothering me. Problems internalized fester and grow to seem insurmountable. On the other hand, once you express them to the outside world they shrivel and seem much more manageable. While once a devotee of the 'ostrich head in the sand' way of life, I now do my best to do the opposite. On this occasion, I chose to blog about how I was feeling.

22 February 2010

Yesterday was a shite day. To be honest, I've been having a lot of shite days recently. Since I was made redundant 10 months ago, the proportion of shite days has increased substantially. Now don't get me wrong, it's not like there's some kind of disaster every day, it's just that I feel like I'm teetering on the spine of a roof and it only takes a tiny bit of wind to make me lose my balance.

I really didn't realize just how much my self-worth was tied up with my work. When I was working full-time I knew my place, I knew my purpose, I felt I was contributing. Now I just feel ... well, kind of lost. And sad. And sorry for myself. So very, very sorry for myself. Some days I feel so sorry for myself I don't even get out of bed. (Haven't said that one out loud before.)

And then of course there's the guilt. Feeling so miserable makes me want to hide away. I feel I don't really have anything to say to people so am more socially uncomfortable than I have ever been. So I'm not keeping in touch with friends. And I feel guilty about that. The only person I am good at keeping in touch with at the moment is my long-suffering boyfriend, who therefore bears the brunt of all of this. He's the one who has to listen to me and watch me dissolve into tears at almost any little thing that goes wrong. So I feel guilty about that. Almost every day I feel I've failed myself in terms of changing my situation, that I haven't emailed or called enough people or made enough of an effort to find a new opportunity. So I feel guilty about that, too.

So it's tough. People are very good; they remind me that this isn't for ever and it will all turn around, and there is a part of me that knows that, but sometimes that part gets drowned out by all the guilt and self-pity. Also, I know that, really, I'm lucky, with no mortgage or children to worry about; things could be so much worse. But that fact can get drowned out as well. I'm also aware that the only person who is going to make my situation better is me. But that seems to be the fact that is buried deepest beneath my personal tragedy on days when things aren't good. On the shite days.

Part of me wants to delete all this; I mean, it's kind of shameful, and not very good PR. But the fact is I'm not the only person going through this. With unemployment at 13.4%, there are lots of us in the same position, so I'm going to be honest and leave it here. I'm having a lot of shite days. But I'm not the only one. And, deep down, I know it's not for ever.

There weren't a huge number of people who were interested in what I had to say, but I shared the post on Facebook and Twitter and people responded to it – enough to make me feel a little bit better – so I decided to make some changes. I was going to get up every day and get dressed. I was going to leave the house, even if it was just to go to the shop. I was going to stop ignoring my friends and, instead, I was going to tell everyone I knew that I really needed work. My pride would have to be put to one side. This sadness had to end. The following month, I got a job! It wasn't my dream job, but it was something to get up for every morning and, really, that was all I needed.

Things to do when you feel like you can't go on

If I'm feeling down, I have a propensity to lie in bed watching endless hours of reality television, but I have found that – unsurprisingly – this doesn't make me feel any better about life. Here is what I do to combat feelings of malaise.

- *Take a shower and get dressed*
  Does anyone feel their best when they've been wearing the same clothes for several days? No.

- *Put on make-up, if that's what you're into*
  This makes me feel really, really good, but I know it's not for everyone.

- *Leave the house*
  Sounds simple, sometimes isn't, but can be, literally, transformative. Even a trip to the supermarket can give a miserable day a lift.

- *Tell someone about it*
  Often, admitting to the dark feelings swirling around your head is the first step to eradicating them. Twitter can be weirdly good for this stuff.

- *Clean your room*
  Really annoying but weirdly beneficial psychologically.

- *Read a book*
  There's something about reading that can help you escape in a way TV just can't; also, you feel smart and productive and, if you're lucky, a little smug.

- **Start something new**

  Blog, paint, write, cook – whatever it is you're into. A feeling of productivity is incredibly valuable.

- **Exercise**

  Okay, okay, it was hard for me even to write, but there's no doubt that a little cycle ride, or even an energetic walk, stirs up something positive in most people. If possible, do it somewhere beautiful, like on a beach or in some woods. If you can't bring yourself to leave the house, try a yoga lesson on YouTube.

- **Forgive yourself**

  Whatever it is you feel like you are failing at currently, let it go. Don't dwell on what you didn't do yesterday; instead, think about what you can do with today.

My own show

In May 2012, 2fm's *Weekend Breakfast* show was in a period of transition, and when I read that the presenters were finishing up I summoned up Ballsy Louise and emailed the man in charge to suggest myself for the slot, subject line: 'Cheeky!'

If I were in this position again, and writing an email like that, I would not be making the subject line 'Cheeky!' I was not being cheeky in asking for an opportunity I was absolutely capable of taking. I had ten years' radio experience and hard work behind me, and I had been doing the occasional show on 2fm for a year and a half, filling in for people, so I knew they were happy with my work. I should not have been apologetic in my approach.

I work hard now to be confident in the way I communicate with people about professional situations, whether that is asking for work or enquiring about overdue payment. If you have something to offer, you have something to offer. You shouldn't devalue yourself by acting like the person at the other end is doing you a favour by even reading your email. That's not to say I have developed a sense of entitlement, but I have worked hard to develop a sense of self-worth and value.

Being overly apologetic is not a mistake that only women make, but I do believe that men, in general, are much more confident about asking for what they want and, frankly, I'm sick of seeing women being passed up for things because they're not as pushy as their male colleagues. Where once I would have been too bashful to indicate what I wanted professionally, I am now very clear about it and take every opportunity to ask for it. It's not always comfortable for me, and it doesn't come naturally, but I honestly believe that, when it comes to work, if you don't ask, you won't get.

I'm sick of seeing women being passed up for things because they're not as pushy as their male colleagues.

I asked, and I got. In his reply to my email the 2fm boss indicated that I was not the first person to contact him about doing the show and that there were people ahead of me in the queue in terms of position

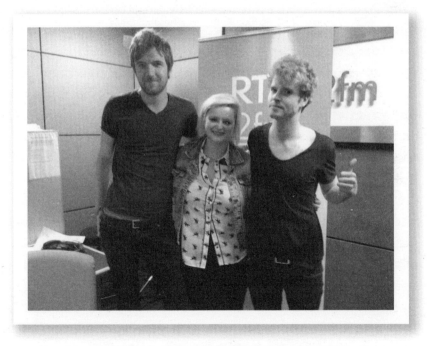

My first time covering for Ryan Tubridy. With Mark and Steve from Kodaline.

and experience in 2fm. However, he asked me to fill in on the show for a few weeks during that transitional period. A few weeks turned out to be almost two years of doing *Weekend Breakfast* every Saturday and Sunday morning, ending only in early 2014, when I got my own nightly show.

My Uncle Greg worked in radio for years when I was younger. He was on pirate radio with a lot of the people you still hear on the air these days and later did some legitimate work on a phone-in show as a producer. I spent a lot of time with him during my visits from America, and I used to love coming up with topics for the show. We used to sit in the back garden together, poring over the papers, discussing what might get people going, and then each night I'd listen in as the topics came to life. I suppose this was my first real radio experience, but I never really thought it was something I'd do as a career.

Years later, when it was looking like radio was going to be my job, Greg warned me off. I couldn't understand it at the time, but now I see exactly where he was coming from. While radio can be lots of fun and very rewarding, if you work as an on-air personality, it lacks any security. There are constant rumours about who is losing their show and who is being moved to one place or another. The newspapers speculate about your job and production staff whisper. When you're part of the production staff with a permanent contract, this gossip can be as much fun as any other office gossip, but when you are the presenter, the rumours are enough to drive you crazy. You feel as though you can't trust anyone and, as much as you like and get along with your bosses, you know they could pull the plug on you at any moment. You'd have to be insane to put yourself in that position, and yet it's the very position I've put myself in.

You have no control over your career as a presenter. It's not like other jobs, where a role becomes available and you are given the opportunity to put yourself forward, to sell yourself as a viable option. Instead, you have to sit quietly, hoping you'll be the chosen one. In many ways, it's hell. You can work for years doing the awkward shifts late at night or early in the morning at the weekend, doing thirteen consecutive early-morning starts over Christmas so that the other presenters can enjoy the season and potentially never see the benefit. You have to be mad to do it, really.

Managing my inner Roy Keane

I've been called a troublemaker more than once during my career. I am the kind of person who finds it hard just to put my head down and get on with it, ignoring whatever's going on around me. If systems aren't working, I find that frustrating. If I have ideas about how things can be better, I want to express them. I'm a bit of a Roy Keane, I suppose: when something's just not good enough, I find it hard to ignore.

However, you can't get away with being a bit of a Roy Keane when you're a woman. A man can demand that things be improved at work and be seen as confident and assertive. When a woman does it, she's often deemed a 'moany cow'. If you're a woman, people don't always want to hear your ideas, and they definitely don't want to hear your complaints. Sometimes, you get lucky and you work with someone who is fully committed to making the organization run as smoothly as possible but, other times, you work with someone who really just wants to do the bare minimum and keep the place afloat. I find these people difficult. I don't ever want just to keep the place afloat. I want the place to be charging across the ocean.

I have experienced the 'moany cow' reaction and the 'troublemaker' reaction and, of course, the 'stupid bitch' reaction. As a result, I have found myself in a strange position in recent years. In spite of being a confident, assertive woman, I became

> *I have experienced the 'moany cow' reaction and the 'troublemaker' reaction and, of course, the 'stupid bitch' reaction.*

afraid to raise my voice. Afraid to complain. Afraid to ask for things at work. If I did manage to ask for something, I would find myself starting my request with an apology. Instead of saying, 'Listen, the computer I edit on isn't working well, I really need a new one,' I would sound pathetic, saying, 'I'm really sorry to bother you, I know you have a lot of work to do and I really wouldn't come to you if it wasn't urgent, but the computer I'm using isn't working very well, so do you think we could have a chat about it sometime?'

Going into meetings with people senior to me, I would find myself nervous and worried about what people might be thinking of me. *Do they think I'm a bitch? Am I too demanding? Am I asking for too much? If I'm too annoying, will they just get rid of me?* I would find myself shrinking back instead of striding forward, prioritizing likeability over asking for what I needed to do my job to the best of my ability.

I hated being like that. Sometimes, I would get annoyed with myself, but then I would realize I hadn't always been this way. I learned to behave like this. I learned via several male superiors who made it clear they didn't want to hear what I had to say. I learned via the guy in my sixth-year English class who shouted, 'Shut up, Louise, no one wants to hear what you have to say!' I learned through experience.

I'm not the only one who struggles with this stuff. I was thrilled to read Jennifer Lawrence's essay for the online newsletter *Lenny* on her experience of sexism at work. Aside from the obvious issue of unequal pay, her reference to the pressure we put on ourselves to be exactly the right female personality at work really rang true for me.

I'm over trying to find the 'adorable' way to state my opinion and still be likeable! Fuck that. I don't think I've ever worked for a man in charge who spent time contemplating what angle he should use to have his voice heard. It's just heard.

punches air

I thought about inequality between the sexes a lot and I realized I wasn't doing myself any favours by trying to wrap myself up as the perfect lady package at work. Not only was I not doing myself any favours, I wasn't doing other women any favours. Like Jennifer, I had to start sucking it up and stop questioning myself. Think like a man, I told myself.

The next time I had a meeting with my boss I made a list of the things I wanted to talk about and, as I walked into the office, I waved it around and laughed. He laughed, too. As I sat down, I looked at my list, fighting the urge to cut it by half at least. Surely I didn't need to bring up all these issues? I didn't want to complain too much. Then the voice in my head said, 'Would a man cut this list in half?' I knew he wouldn't, so I stuck to my guns and brought up all the items on my list.

You're not going to believe it, but it was grand! My boss made notes of the issues I was raising, and we ended the meeting on good terms. If I had trusted my instincts, then I would still be frustrated over the things I had decided not to mention. Now, I find myself saying both to myself and to female friends, 'What would a man do? Would a man be afraid of this? Would a man be concerned about asking for a well-deserved pay rise? Would a man be afraid to suggest a new system?' I have found it to be incredibly empowering.

Having said that, not everyone will have success with this method. There are a lot of sexists out there in our workplaces who do not want to hear what women have to say.

(There are also a lot of dickhead bosses who do not want to hear what anyone has to say.) However, I don't think that means you should silence yourself. I think maybe you should find another job or complain to their superior, but you should not silence yourself. The more we, as women, edit ourselves and try to mould ourselves into the perfect little woman at work, the more we'll be treated like 'women' and the less like equals. We are just as smart as men, just as deserving as them and just as hard-working as them, so we deserve just as much power and airtime. Let's not let ourselves down by not asking for it.

The best place I've ever worked was also the one where the gender balance was most even. It was amazing to go to work and feel respected and heard. I was able to raise issues, and they were listened to thoughtfully and considerately. Where suggestions were fair, they were implemented; where they were not, they were discussed thoroughly. People's time was respected, and the fact that they had lives outside work. As a result, the staff was committed and hard-working. The company made an effort to hire people who would get along, so communication at work was easy and fun. I felt a real sense of belonging. It's incredible how little things like feeling valued as an employee can alter your attitude to your workplace. It's shocking that so many companies seem to overlook this.

4
Cancer

My mystery illness

It all started on 30 November 2013. That Saturday night before we went out, I felt a bit off. I had always viewed my good health as something to be proud of and commented to my friends that it was very unlike me to be sick. I decided to go ahead with my night out, though, refusing to be one of those 'weak, sick people' (as I secretly thought of them). Well, frankly, I was being an idiot. By the end of the weekend, after a lot of running around between a doctor who was on call in north Dublin and the A&E department of the Mater, I'd had my appendix out. The medics told Gordon it had been a close call. Apparently, my appendix had been seriously inflamed, and they couldn't believe I had been as well as I had. All along, I had thought it was some gastric problem and had been popping Deflatines.

I don't tell you this to try to convince you of how big and brave I am (although, obviously, I'm a very brave girl – that goes without saying: *winky smiley*) but to explain how that experience made me distrust my body. If I had felt relatively fine during acute appendicitis, then could I believe the signals my body gave me at all?

The operation was the start of eight months of worsening health. First, I had a post-surgery abscess. Then it seemed like my body was going into early menopause. My energy levels plummeted. Unusually for me, so did my appetite. I was back and forth to the Mater regularly. The doctors were mystified. One of the blood tests they took indicated that my body was fighting infection, but it wasn't clear where from. I was passed from one department of the hospital to another.

It's hard for me to have any real perspective on this, because I was so convinced that I was fine for the duration of what I laughingly referred to as my 'mystery illness'. Later, Gordon pointed it out that I slowly became a very sick person. I was still going to work every day, but I rarely lasted past eleven on a night out. I fell asleep on the couch every evening, and my mood was suffering, too. I attributed all this to a busy work schedule and started seeing a personal trainer in the hope that exercise would bring me the magical energy people who do it always go on about.

I was having weekly blood tests and weigh-ins, and my weight was rapidly decreasing. I, of course, was delighted to see the number on the scale going down and horrified when Dr Mallon, the consultant in the Infectious Diseases clinic, told me he needed to see it going up. My entire life, doctors had been telling me to lose weight, and now, when I was spending a fortune on a personal trainer and seeing some results, I was supposed to undo my hard work?! The thing is, if I had been honest with myself, I would have realized the weight loss wasn't a result of the personal training. My appetite had just disappeared: I had no interest in food and was eating very little.

My entire life, doctors had been telling me to lose weight, and now, when I was spending a fortune on a personal trainer and seeing some results, I was supposed to undo my hard work?!

By August 2014 I was having a ball in work. I was filling in for Ryan Tubridy for a fortnight, doing the type of show I absolutely love, where I get to do interviews and interact with the public. The mystery illness was just an annoying thing I had to deal with on the side. Yes, I was tired, and no, I didn't feel a hundred per cent, but if they just figured it out I'd be grand. I was really looking forward to going on holiday. So I was gutted when I developed a very bad pain in my side which wouldn't go away.

I rang my dad, miserably, and asked him what I should do. I really wanted to go away, and I knew he'd tell me what the right thing to do was. He'd raised us to be tough: we were not people who called in sick. We toughed things out.

'Will you be able to enjoy yourself as you are at the moment?' he asked.

I knew then that I couldn't go. I rang Jane, one of the doctors on Dr Mallon's team in the Mater, and we agreed that I would have to be admitted. I needed proper tests to get to the bottom of whatever was going on.

I was ragin'. This whole thing had gone on for so long, and I was convinced I was fine. It seemed like such a rigmarole over nothing. I spent a week in the hospital, having tests, one leading to another. I felt like a fool in the ward, with people who I considered to be genuinely sick. I felt like I was taking up the bed of someone who was in genuine need. 'That woman has *cancer*!' I'd say to Gordon. 'I shouldn't be here.' I felt like I should apologize to the nurses and carers for wasting their time.

The tests culminated in a biopsy on one of my lymph nodes. I had some growths on my spleen, apparently, and an enlarged lymph node on my left-hand side, so they wanted to check it out. I won't lie: an alarm bell rang when I heard the words 'lymph nodes'. I'd watched a hell of a lot of *ER* and *Grey's Anatomy*, and something told me this wouldn't be good. But – ever the compartmentalizer – I pushed those thoughts to one side and was delighted to be released with an appointment to come back and get the results the following week.

Since I was meant to be in San Sebastián on holiday, I enjoyed the days I had scheduled to be off. People at work encouraged me to take whatever time I needed. Again, I was waiting to be caught out, convinced that, when it turned out to be nothing, everyone would laugh and roll their eyes at what a drama queen I had been. Alarm bells rang for a second time when I got a phone call from one of the doctors on the team, calling to make sure I was coming in to get my biopsy results. Why would a doctor call to confirm an appointment? If it was just a run-of-the-mill confirmation, wouldn't a member of the administrative staff have called? Again, I swept these thoughts to one side.

When Gordon announced that he was going to come with me to my appointment, I argued with him. It seemed unnecessary. After all, I had gone to all the others on my own. He insisted, though, and when the morning came and alarm bells rang for a third time, I was glad he was with me. I was back in Dr Mallon's clinic, and when he crossed the waiting room I felt he was avoiding my gaze. Something was up.

When I was called almost immediately, I knew it was bad news. I knew it was bad news when he took us into a different room than normal. I knew it was bad news because Jane wasn't there. Jane had always been there, and we'd always engaged in a bit of banter. I was scared.

He said it very well. 'All through our investigation we have been trying to rule out the possibility of lymphoma and, unfortunately, we haven't been able to.'

I knew what that meant. It meant cancer. It meant that I had cancer.

For a minute, all the things you think you know about cancer if you don't know anything about it flashed through my mind. I thought about sitting with a blanket over my lap. I pictured myself bald. I thought about dying. Then my brain went into preservation mode and all I wanted to know was what we were going to do about this. I just wasn't going to consider that this might be something I wouldn't be able to get over. Fortunately, Dr Mallon seemed to think this was something I could get over, too.

He told me that Hodgkin's was a rare cancer that occurred most frequently in young people. He assured me that this form of cancer responded really well to chemo and that because I was young and fit I was in a very strong position for treatment. I have to tell you that, even in the midst of being diagnosed with cancer, I got a real thrill when he referred to me as fit. It was the first time in my life a doctor – or indeed any human – had said such a thing about me.

Anyway, once I got over the 'fit' thrill, I tuned back into the conversation. He was talking about the chemotherapy I would be having. 'Chemotherapy,' I said, over and over, in my head. 'Cancer.'

Dr Mallon assured me that the team who would be treating me was the best of the best, and that the consultant I was being referred to was super. They wanted to see me the next day, but he was going to go away and double-check the time.

I don't know if he really needed to double-check the time or if he was just giving Gordon and me a little bit of space to take in what we'd just been told. When he left the room, I cried silently while Gordon tried to comfort me. I

I cried silently while Gordon tried to comfort me. I batted him away. I didn't want to be touched or comforted, I just wanted to be tough.

batted him away. I didn't want to be touched or comforted, I just wanted to be tough. I *was* tough, and I was going to beat this; that was just how it was going to be. Dr Mallon was gone for what felt like ages, while Gordon and I sat there looking at each other, me occasionally saying, 'Cancer,' incredulously. I couldn't believe it.

By the time Dr Mallon came back, I wanted to get out of there. I needed to be alone to process what was going on, to have some space to have an actual reaction rather than attempting to hold it together because I was in public. He gave me a yellow appointment card and wrote his email address on it, explaining that they wouldn't have any need to see me in the Infectious Diseases clinic any more but if at any stage at all I had any questions about anything that was going on with my treatment I shouldn't hesitate to contact him. I was really touched by that at the time, and I'm still touched by it now. I never needed to contact him, but it was so great to know that I had the option of a familiar and trust-worthy person on the receiving end of an email.

Gordon and I were in a daze when we walked out of the clinic that day, through the busy waiting room. 'Lucky feck-ers,' Gordon muttered to me under his breath.

'This is an HIV clinic. Some of them probably aren't very lucky,' I replied, on autopilot.

We walked home in shock, me saying, out loud, 'I have cancer,' again and again.

Boarding the cancer train

What do you do when you've just been told you have cancer? For an age, we just sat in our apartment in silence, unsure of what to do. I decided to call my dad, but I struggled to get the words out. I wept on the phone to him as he did his best to say the right things.

I was due to see my entire family that evening for my sister's birthday dinner, but I didn't want to do a big, dramatic announcement at the table so I felt it was only right to let them know ahead of time. I did not, however, want to weep down the phone to all of them. It wasn't fair. So I took a deep breath and went about the phone calls in a different way. It was clear that, to avoid upset, I needed to lead with the good news. Yes, I had cancer, but it was very treatable, and I was going to be fine. I smiled as I said the words, hoping that whoever was on the other end of the phone line would believe me, because I knew any upset on their part would only set me off. It worked! They all reacted pragmatically, if a little doubtfully, largely saying, 'Well, that sounds okay, if you're sure.' My mom was the funniest. After the months of me being ill and her watching the weight drop off me, she had clearly convinced herself that I had a terminal illness, because her relief was palpable. She sounded positively delighted at this turn of events. 'It's treatable! That's *great*!' I couldn't stop laughing over it. How many people's mothers react with delight when they're told their kid has cancer? For once, her tendency to fear and assume the worst worked in our favour.

I only made two other phone calls outside of my immediate family. One was to my best mate, and one was to Dan Healy, the head of 2fm. I didn't know what the story was with work and treatment, but I couldn't stay off interminably without offering some explanation. He could not have been more supportive, which was a relief. After that, I didn't want to speak to anyone else. I decided to keep the diagnosis to myself until I knew what was to come. Our family dinner that night was bizarre. We tried our best to be normal, as I joked about stealing Úna's birthday thunder, but I had a single statement running around my head on a loop. 'I have cancer, I have cancer, I have cancer . . .' I had cancer.

> *I had a single statement running around my head on a loop. 'I have cancer, I have cancer, I have cancer . . .' I had cancer.*

My younger sister, Aoife, asked me if I was scared. I told her I was, and it was the truth. All I knew about chemotherapy was what I'd seen in films and on television and, let's be honest, they never really portray it as a walk in the park. I wasn't afraid I was going to die, though, and I told her as much. There was no way I was even going to consider that as a possibility.

I woke up the next day with a jolt, enjoying that bleary moment you have in the morning before you remember what's going on in your life or what you have to do that day. It didn't last, and a few minutes later I was sitting on the toilet, crying. 'I have cancer. I have cancer. I have cancer.'

Later that morning Gordon and I stepped out of the lift on the seventh floor of the Mater Hospital and into the waiting area for St Vincent's Ward for the first time. I'll be honest, I was horrified. We sat in the waiting area for ages, which gave us plenty of time to take in the information pamphlets on dealing with symptoms and the ads for wig shops. There were signs on the wall for the Daffodil Centre, a place in the hospital where cancer patients could get support, and various other support groups. 'I get it,' I said to Gordon. 'I have cancer. Do they really need to shove it down my throat?' As we sat there, a woman wearing a headscarf arrived. She sat down beside us and opened her book, waiting to be called for treatment. I found it hard not to stare. She was a cancer patient. I was going to be like her. I had cancer.

We were ushered into the ward itself and I found myself confronted with the sight of people being given chemotherapy. It looked just as it did on TV: people sitting in armchairs, hooked up to drips. They were cancer patients. I was going to be like them. I had cancer.

By the time I got to the room in which I was going to meet my doctor and have a bone-marrow biopsy, I was shaking. The friendly specialist haematology nurse, who had welcomed us warmly, asked me to update her on what was going on, but I couldn't get the words out and instead immediately started crying. I was overwhelmed. Gordon spoke for me and, fortunately, Sinéad, the nurse, was the type who sympathized but did not mollycoddle, so I managed to pull myself together.

Soon we were joined by Dr Fortune, the consultant haematologist who would be overseeing my case. She gave me all the information. I was going to have chemotherapy every two weeks for approximately six months. I was almost certainly going to lose my hair. Usually, the kind of chemo I was going to receive was not too hard on female fertility, but they were going to give me an injection that would reduce the risk further. That sounded fine to me. I didn't give my fertility any more thought. I might feel sick but I wouldn't necessarily vomit. I might get mouth sores. I would have to be very careful to avoid infections. I wasn't allowed to travel. I should avoid unpasteurized cheese and eat only vacuum-packed meat.

But could I go to Electric Picnic? They laughed. I was starting chemo the following Tuesday and I wanted to know if I could get to my favourite festival. 'That'll have to be your last hurrah,' Sinéad said.

I had my bone-marrow biopsy and, fortunately, the lymphoma had not made its way in there. I was handed another yellow appointment card and some leaflets, and told not to google my diagnosis. They would see me on Tuesday. With that, I was a ticket-holding passenger on the cancer train.

Chemo zombie

Cancer patients on TV seem to vomit endlessly, sobbing on the bathroom floor as the people in their lives desert them. I was sure the people in my life weren't going to desert me, but I was worried about the vomiting. As a result, I emailed a guy I knew from Twitter who I knew had had Hodgkin's and asked him to give me the scoop. What was it really going to be like?

His reply was incredible. I was a relative stranger, but he took the time to tell me of his chemo experience in great detail. He outlined the process step by step, and I was pleasantly surprised at what I learned. He told me that he had made it through his entire treatment without being sick, which came as a huge relief to me. No one likes to vomit, and that was the thing I was most afraid of. In fact, he told me, there were great drugs these days which dealt with almost all the side effects of chemo. *Take the drugs*, he said. I laughed. He was right.

As a result of his email, I felt reasonably confident when I headed into my first session. Judging by what he'd told me, and some stuff I'd read online (I know, I know, I promise I didn't google too much), the first session tended to be pretty easy. From what I had read, chemo was cumulative, and the impact on your body grew as treatment went on, so, as a result, I should be fine on Day 1. I was a little nervous, but Gordon was allowed to come with me and we smiled our way through it, joking with the nurses and taking everything in.

When we left the hospital I felt a little rough. I was really cold and very tired, and by the time I got home I didn't even have the energy to take my clothes off, passing out instead on top of the covers in our bedroom. Gordon decided to go to work for a few hours while I was asleep, and when he got home at around eight that evening I was still asleep. When I woke up I had a terrible headache, and we took my temperature with our newly purchased thermometer. We were under strict instructions that if my temperature reached a certain level we needed to ring the hospital immediately. It was well above, and the haematologist on call told us to go to A&E. I was furious. I don't remember having a strop too many times during the whole cancer thing, but I definitely had a strop that night. The first day was meant to be okay! I was meant to feel fine! I was prepared to feel rubbish down the line, but it wasn't meant to happen yet!

The first day was meant to be okay! I was meant to feel fine! I was prepared to feel rubbish down the line, but it wasn't meant to happen yet!

We made our way to A&E, where the haematologist met us and took some blood. At this stage I had given so much blood I felt like it could feed a vampire colony. After about an hour the doctor came back and said she was happy that what had happened was a reaction to one of the anti-sickness drugs they had given me and not anything more sinister. Off we went on our not-so-merry way.

The next time I went for treatment they changed the anti-sickness drug they'd given me because of my dodgy reaction to it. This time, I was at the hospital on my own, feeling very brave indeed. My appetite had recently returned and I was feeling better than I had in ages. I settled into my chair as they gave me the anti-sickness drug, thinking of the cheese sandwich I was going to have when the cart came around. I might feel a bit snoozy with this drug, the nurse warned, and soon enough I nodded off. I woke up a few times over the course of the next couple of hours, but I couldn't keep my eyes open. However, I was aware of a change in the way I was feeling. When the cart came around I couldn't stomach the thought of a sandwich, and by the time I left the hospital that evening I knew something was amiss.

With hindsight, I probably should have turned around and gone back inside, but at the time I just wanted to go home after spending hours in the hospital. I lived on Capel Street, about five minutes in a cab or a fifteen-minute walk from the hospital. I didn't trust myself to make it the five minutes in the cab without needing to throw up, so I decided to walk home.

I walked as quickly as I could. I felt like I was in a haze; my vision was blurred and saliva was pooling in my mouth as I tried not to puke. 'Just get home, just get home, just get home,' I chanted in my head. I managed to make it to our apartment building, half crawling, half running up the stairs, before falling into the bathroom and vomiting for the first of around seventy times over the course of the next six hours. Between bursts of vomiting, I lay on the bathroom floor, genuinely afraid. I felt drugged, which I had been, but this didn't feel right. I couldn't see properly, or stand. For the first time in my life, I rang my mother when I was sick. I had always been entirely self-sufficient but, this time, I needed reassurance that I was going to be okay. When she didn't answer, I wept, calling Gordon and barely managing to get the words 'Come home' out of my mouth.

By the time he got home I had given up on the bathroom.

Everything that had been inside me was now out, so what had been uncontrollable vomiting had become uncontrollable heaving instead. A plastic bin beside the soft bed seemed like a wiser option than lying on the floor of the bathroom. I can't imagine the fright Gordon must have got when he found me hanging off the side of the bed with my head over the bin, my body convulsing. I had asked him to come home but now I couldn't handle having him anywhere near me, so he was forced into the sitting room, where he sat on the couch, worrying and listening to the sounds of my sickness, jumping up to run in to me every time he heard a new bout of heaving begin. In the end, I told him not to bother.

There was nothing he could do. There was nothing I could do. I just had to lie there and wait for it to be over. At long last, I fell asleep, waking up now and again to heave, and around midnight it stopped. It was the worst physical trauma I had ever experienced.

The next day the vomiting had stopped, but I was still nauseous and found the only way to keep that at bay was to eat. It seemed counterintuitive, but crackers and toast seemed to quell the feeling of my stomach turning, so I snacked all day. By the third day, I felt significantly better and found myself looking back on the previous day's ordeal with fear. I didn't know if I could handle it happening again. Aside from the actual discomfort of heaving for hours on end, the experience had been frightening. What if it was going to be like this every time? I knew it shouldn't be, but what if it was?

By the time I went back to the hospital for my third treatment, I was terrified. I began to feel nauseous when I arrived. A nurse went through the usual questions with me before I was given chemo. Any pins and needles? Any temperatures? Any vomiting? I laughed, bitterly, at that question. Yes, I said,

'Lots.' 'How many times?' she asked. Again, I laughed, and explained that it had been beyond counting. 'Sixty? Seventy?' She seemed shocked. A doctor came to speak to me and she explained that they would be trying something new. This time, she said, this time, the side effects wouldn't be so bad. I said that I was feeling nauseous, and she told me this was quite common after a traumatic episode like I'd had. It was all in my head – pre-emptive nausea.

That day I found myself sharing a chemo room with a woman who was chatty and full of life, and she distracted me from my fear. We sat, hooked up to our individual drips, and chatted until she told me she was about to fall asleep, and would I mind if she did? I didn't at all. While she slept, I felt my stomach turn. It was happening again. I was panicky, and worried, but I convinced myself that it was my imagination. It was just because I was so afraid. I was making it up.

This time I had taken precautions to ensure that I wouldn't be alone after chemo. My dad was waiting for me outside in his car, and as I left the hospital I rang him to tell him that I was going to be sick and we needed to get home pronto. I didn't even make it to the first set of traffic lights before I had to open the car door to vomit on to the street. There was little in my stomach, so for the rest of the journey I heaved into my scarf, apologizing to my dad and telling him I wasn't going to get anything on his car. I don't think I've ever seen him so scared. I couldn't control the convulsions. By the time we got home I could barely speak and went straight into my bedroom with the bin, closing the door behind me and bunkering down for the hours of hell ahead of me.

Gordon came home an hour later and found my dad sitting in silence in the sitting room and me in a daze in the bedroom. At one stage, the heaving was so intense that I had an accident in my pyjama bottoms. I called Gordon from the bathroom, asking him to bring me new ones. It was at this point that I knew our relationship would never be the same.

All boundaries were nullified. Once you have to call your boyfriend to assist you because you have shat in your pyjamas, everything is different. In fairness to him, he didn't blink an eye.

> *Once you have to call your boyfriend to assist you because you have shat in your pyjamas, everything is different.*

I stayed in my bedroom waiting for the pain to end, while my dad insisted on buying Gordon a takeaway and remaining with him for a few hours. I've never asked him why, but I can only assume he didn't want to leave him alone in such a horrendous situation. When I look back, I think that day was the lowest point. I was so incredibly sick, and no one could help me. I saw fear on my dad's face, and how desperately Gordon wanted to help. I had become the cancer person on TV or in the movies, the very thing I had been afraid of.

You can imagine how I felt when I returned to the hospital for my fourth treatment. I begged to be given the anti-sickness drug from Week 1. I could take the headache! Anything to avoid the vomiting. My dad collected me from the hospital that day, and I gingerly got into his car and explained that I *thought* I was okay. He had stocked the passenger side of the car with airplane sick-bags decorated with smiley faces, just in case. Fortunately, they were unnecessary. I made it home and into the apartment without incident. As I realized that it wasn't going to happen this time, I felt positively elated. When Gordon walked in the door I was sitting on the couch watching TV. 'NO PUKING!' I shouted, hands in the air. His face was covered in pure delight. I even managed to eat that night, as we revelled in the simple joy of me being an actual human as opposed to the chemo zombie I had been the last few weeks.

Luckily, that was the end of my career as a chemo zombie. I didn't vomit a single other time throughout my treatment, and generally avoided nausea entirely. When I think about the rest of the course of chemo, I feel like I sailed through it, though that's not entirely true. Chemo is really hard on your body, and some of the side effects are really unpleasant. At times I had extreme pains in my bones and there was little they could do to help. I had a manky taste in my mouth constantly. I had absolutely no sex drive. Towards the end of my treatment, I was wiped out, as the tiredness built. It wasn't easy. However, after the vomiting, the most difficult thing for me to deal with was the constipation.

Prior to my experience with it, I would have assumed constipation wasn't a big deal. I mean, how bad could it be? The answer is, absolutely terrible. After a couple of months of chemo and various other drugs, I was really struggling to go to the toilet. Just in case you don't know, if you don't manage to do a big job in the toilet when you need to, the big job gets harder, in both senses of the word. Every time I managed to go, it was a massive struggle. It was painful, there was tearing – it was hell. I found myself afraid to leave the house at times because I knew that if I felt like I might be able to, or need to, use the loo, I wouldn't want to be anywhere but home.

I tried everything I could. I drank as much stool softener and prune juice as I could, dosed myself up on Dulcolax, double-dropped medically prescribed laxatives. Nothing seemed to help. One night I woke up with the need upon me and, while I struggled on the toilet, I wept and shivered. I spent the next two hours going from bed to the toilet and getting nowhere. Around 4 a.m., I crawled back into bed, shaking and pressing into Gordon for warmth, wrung out from the ordeal. He wanted to call the hospital but I couldn't face the idea of having to go somewhere. However, when I woke up the next morning my temperature was high, so we went straight to A&E. As it turned out, I had an infection. I was checked in to St Vincent's Ward in the Mater and spent a few days there. The infection itself was cleared quickly, but they were reluctant to let me leave without me having had a successful bowel movement. I literally spent the next couple of days in hospital trying to poop, while my mates made jokes about me being hospitalized for being 'full of shit'. I did my best to encourage my body by walking rings around the hospital and eating fruit to beat the band. Every time I wandered by the nurses' station my lovely nurse Amy would ask, 'Anything?' 'Nope,' I would say sadly.

Eventually, a phosphate enema managed to get things going a little bit. And this is the bit where I tell you that cancer really does everything it can to reduce you to your most abject level. There is nothing like presenting your bare arse to a nurse, after days of discussing the intimate details of your bowels with her, to make you lose any semblance of pride. I had always been an open book, but now it seemed there was literally nothing that wasn't up for discussion.

I spent the rest of my chemo time comparing constipation stories with a pal in the UK who happened to be having chemo at the same time. We had been friendly before, but now we were *friends* – poop sisters, if you will. It was great to talk about it with someone who understood, which is why I've gone on about it at such length here. Constipation is a side effect of many illnesses and associated treatments and, if you don't have someone to discuss it with, it can be very isolating and lonely. I'm here to tell you that you're not alone. If you find yourself in this shitty situation (see what I did there?), pick someone in your life to vent to about it; otherwise, you'll lose your mind. You may be embarrassed, but I'm sure there is someone who will understand and be willing to commiserate with you. If there isn't, then I think you should (a) tweet or email me, and (b) get better friends. 💩

Twelve things never to say to someone who has cancer*

1. ***That's a good cancer to have.***
   There are no good cancers. There are definitely some which respond better to treatment than others, and I'm allowed to observe that as the patient, but you are not.

   Please don't tell me how lucky I am. I may not be in the humour to hear it.

2. ***Cancer isn't as hard as it used to be.***
   That's funny, because it felt pretty tough this morning, when I was lying on the bathroom floor weeping over a bowel movement.

3. ***I've always wanted to shave my head.***
   Losing your hair to chemo is not the same as shaving your head because you thought Natalie Portman looked cool in *V for Vendetta*.

4. ***You look like Natalie Portman in* V for Vendetta!**
   No, I don't.

5. ***We didn't think you'd be up for it.***
   Don't assume we're not able to do things just because we have cancer. Keep inviting us to stuff. Sometimes we won't be up to it, but sometimes we will, and we desperately need to leave the house.

* First published on BuzzFeed, February 2015.

6. *You're so brave.*
    We know you mean well when you say this, but we don't feel brave. Bravery is something that happens when someone chooses to take on something scary. We don't have a choice.

7. *Have you tried . . .?*
    Unless you have a piece of advice so stellar you think we literally can't go on without it, please don't make suggestions about our treatment. Yes, eating kiwis may be an effective way of combating constipation in your everyday life, but if the industrial-strength, medical-grade laxatives an actual doctor has prescribed for me aren't working, then adding more fruit to my diet probably won't either.

8. *If anyone can beat this, you can.*
    Because people who die as a result of cancer didn't fight hard enough?

9. *Remember, there's always someone worse off than you.*
    So helpful.

10. *I know how you feel.*
    No, you don't.

11. *At least you'll have loads of free time now.*
    I am not on holiday. I have taken time off work because dealing with cancer is, literally, a full-time job.

12. Congratulations! You're done!

It's not necessarily over just because we've had our last scheduled bit of chemo or radiation.

Reaching the end of treatment can be a really scary time, so let me tell you when I'm ready to celebrate.

So what should you say?

I don't really know what to say.

It's okay for you to be honest about how you're feeling. We don't expect you to be an expert in dealing with this really tough situation.

I'm sorry you're going through this.

Sometimes, a simple acknowledgement that things are a bit crap right now really helps.

Do you need a lift home from chemo?

Specific offers of help are much better than the general 'I'm here if you need me' type. We'll actually take you up on them, and they will genuinely make a difference.

Have you seen . . .?

Movie and telly recommendations are invaluable for days when we can't get off the couch and feel like we've exhausted Netflix.

Bald

One of the first things I thought of when I was diagnosed with cancer was my hair. Hair loss is so synonymous with cancer, I can't imagine there are many women who wouldn't immediately start picturing themselves bald. I was particularly irritated at the prospect of losing my hair because I had been growing it for months. I am not the type to have naturally long, luscious hair – my attention span is far too short and I enjoy the drama of a big change too much for that. I was the kind of person who would shave half her head for the thrill of it, or dye her hair purple on a whim. However, I wanted to have the option of long hair for my wedding, and my hairdresser had told me that, if I continued bleaching it, it would never grow. So during the period before my diagnosis, my hair had been a boring, almost natural colour. I hated it, but I had begrudgingly accepted it. It had grown long enough for it to be in a cute little ponytail when I found out I was going to lose it.

It's the chemo that does it, and my consultant told me almost everyone who receives my type of chemo loses their hair. (Not every type results in hair loss. In fact, I had to commiserate with a friend that she was *not* going to lose her hair during the type of chemo she was receiving: 'I'm not even going to get the drama of it!' she said. Cancer jokes are important.) The reason you lose your hair is that chemo attacks your fastest-growing cells. Cancer cells, cells in your mouth, your nails, all this kind of craic. Anything fast-growing would be

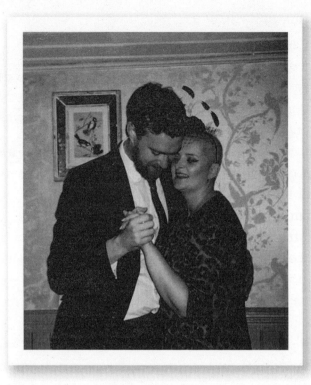

*At a wedding with Gordon in
November 2014. Wearing
a wig was not for me.*

affected, and my hair was going to say goodbye. When I left that day I rang my hairdresser immediately.

'We need to dye my hair pink, and we need to do it as quickly as possible!' I said, having demanded to speak to him personally when I had failed to convince the receptionist.

'But Louise! All your hard work! We can't bleach it again!'

'It's just that . . . It just . . . It doesn't really . . . Okay, I'm just going to say it. I have cancer, and I'm about to lose my hair, and while I have it I want it to be pink.'

'Come in tomorrow,' he said. And I did.

My hair was gloriously pink, like candy. Between it and my

cancer-thin body I felt like a total babe. Alas, it was not to last. It's different for everyone, but I started to notice my hair going after around my third treatment. I was sitting on the couch, watching telly, when I ran my fingers through my hair and some came out. Not a dramatic clump, but a few strands. I did it again. A few

My hair was gloriously pink, like candy. Between it and my cancer-thin body I felt like a total babe.

more. After a few more tests I showed Gordon. I felt a strange combination of excitement and doom. As I've said, I do love a dramatic hair change, but this was real cancer stuff and I wasn't sure if I was able for it.

All the advice I'd been given had said that, once your hair starts to go, you should get rid of it all. Otherwise, you're facing a tortuous, gradual descent into baldness, or else you'll wake up one morning and it will all be left on your pillow.

Christian Shannon of Brown Sugar in Dublin has been trained specifically in the art of caring for cancer patients' hair, and he had already offered his services, so I got in touch with him and arranged to have my hair shaved off a few days later. It was going to be grand. I was going to be grand.

On the day of the appointment I went to get my eyebrows done, thinking that if I had no hair they would be very important. The kind woman in the salon asked me what we were doing. As I tried to explain, I started crying, and I didn't stop until she was finished. As I lay there in the chair, tears streaming down my face, I just couldn't believe this was all happening to me. I couldn't believe I had cancer. I couldn't believe I was about to have my head shaved. I just couldn't believe it.

125

Gordon and my best mate Sarah were coming with me for the shave, so I pulled myself together after the eyebrows. This was the first thing the camera was filming for the documentary as well, so I felt it was important to be brave. Those shots ended up being the opening scene in the documentary, and now when I watch them they make me unbelievably sad. It's so obvious to me that I was faking it, but on the day I really convinced myself that it was all okay. It's a classic Louise move to think that if I say it's okay, and act like it's okay, it will be okay. It works for a while but, in time, it all comes crashing down.

I left the salon wearing a wig I'd bought on the advice of the hospital. I didn't think I wanted one, but the experts had told me I should get one just in case I found myself feeling awkward about being bald. I had rushed the buying process, uncomfortable with it all and eager for it to be over. It was a nice wig, and Christian styled it beautifully, but I hated it. It felt fake to me, and one thing I am not is fake. I am uncomfortable pretending to be something I'm not, which gets me into trouble a lot of the time. (I can't, for example, pretend to be happy when I'm unhappy – not a good characteristic at work or in awkward social situations. I can't ever successfully pretend to like someone who I don't like, so sometimes I come across as a bit of a bitch. Fortunately, I like the vast majority of people.)

I found the idea of wearing a wig awful. I didn't want to cover up what I was experiencing, and I didn't feel like I should have to.

As a result of this compulsion to be sincere, I found the idea of wearing a wig awful. I didn't want to cover up what I was experiencing, and I didn't feel like I should have to. Also, I am a very warm person and sweaty at the best of times, and if you put a wig on me I will melt faster than you can say 'Wicked Witch of the West'. The wig was not for me, and I whipped it off after leaving the salon. I was convinced everyone was staring at me, but I had Gordon and Sarah with me so I bravely carried on. The next day I posted a photo on Instagram with the chipper caption, 'Hair today, gone tomorrow.' I was grand!

I was grand until the following day when Gordon was at work and I needed to go to Tesco and I found myself

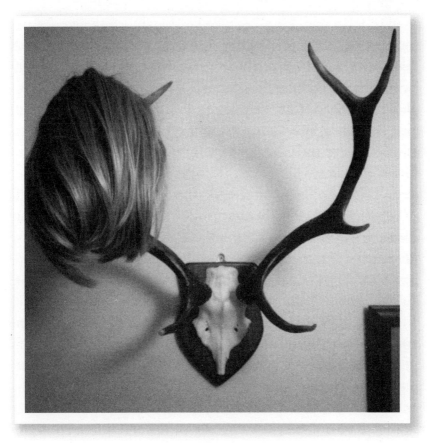

The best place for the wig!

paralysed, unable to leave the house. I felt sure that if I went outside people would stare at me, and not in the way I liked. I felt that people would know immediately that I had cancer. I felt I had lost my femininity. I felt annoyed that I had allowed myself to link my femininity to something as superficial as hair. I felt shallow, and petty. I felt scared. I cried my eyes out. Now I understood why people wore wigs.

After a while, I pulled myself together and went to the shop. It was fine. No one stared. I started pottering around town on my good days. Sometimes I wore a hat, but most of the time it didn't stay on long because of the sweating. I got used to it. In fact, I kind of liked it. I just looked like one of those badass women who chooses to shave her head because WHY THE FUCK NOT! My feelings changed, however, when I caught a glimpse of the top of my head one day in a changing room. It didn't look shaved any more. It looked thin and sick. I cried again. I rang Gordon. I panicked. I felt like I couldn't leave the changing room. When I got home, I got Gordon to help me shave my head again, this time with a clean blade.

As it turned out, I had to shave my head lots of times throughout treatment. I never lost all of my hair; about thirty per cent of it continued to grow. Enough that I had to keep it in check, but not enough that it didn't look awful if it was any length at all. By the end of treatment I was a total pro with the clippers and had come to terms with having a haircut that matched my dad's.

In fact, it was the eyebrows and eyelashes which hurt the most. The hair I could style out with androgynous clothes and cool hats, but if you lose your eyebrows and eyelashes – well, that's a dead giveaway. You're sick, no doubt about it.

Having said that, there's a lot you can do with make-up,

and I experimented, finding products that worked for me and figuring out a way to cover up the appearance of having cancer. Not that there's anything wrong with looking like you have cancer – to each their own. I just didn't want the first thing people thought when they saw me to be *cancer*! I think I succeeded.

I shaved my head for the last time in March 2015, one month after my last chemotherapy treatment. Well, I say it was the last time; I haven't ruled out doing it again for recreational purposes. It's been great to watch my hair grow. I love running my fingers through it and looking in the mirror to find that I look like someone who chose a hairstyle instead of having one inflicted upon them. The longer it gets, the more the cancer will seem like a distant memory, I think, and it's nice to have a physical reminder of the distance.

Clear!

I wake up covered in sweat on the couch two days before my scan. I haven't had chemo in weeks but the hot flushes have not gone away. However, this one feels frighteningly reminiscent of the sweats I started having ten months ago. The sweats that led me to go to my GP in the first place.

I've been telling everyone for weeks now that I feel grand, and I do, but then I thought I felt grand right before I was diagnosed, too. I've been saying that all the symptoms I have feel like chemo symptoms rather than cancer symptoms, which is also true, but then I had this sweat. And now I'm thinking about the sweats I had yesterday in the pub. Were they chemo sweats or were they cancer sweats? I'm scared.

I haven't really been scared lately. Yes, there were moments of fear immediately following my diagnosis but, if I'm honest, my brain swept them to one side and refused to let me consider any outcome that wasn't complete and total recovery after six months of chemo. There was the day I became a chemo zombie for the first time, lying on the cold floor of my bathroom in a haze; I was definitely scared then. But, honestly, that has been it.

Now I'm sitting on my couch, realizing there's a possibility that there are cancer cells multiplying inside me with every moment. It's possible that my scan won't be clear. It's possible that I'll have to postpone my life all over again.

Gordon and I agreed in the days after my diagnosis that we would be honest with each other about our feelings. I didn't want there to be a situation where he was upset or angry and I didn't know about it. He said the same. I upheld my part of the bargain, but he recently confessed that he had not. There had been difficult moments I didn't know about. I hate that. But now I find myself thinking that I can't share this fear with him. We're so close, so nearly there, and I have made it this far without ever being scared. Surely I can fake it for a few more days? Surely I won't ruin my run of strength now? Surely I can be stoic?

I found out the good news in the airport. I was sitting in the bar with my whole family, waiting to take off on a 'sun holiday'. (The first time we'd ever gone away together . . . it rained non-stop.) I recognized the hospital's phone number on my mobile straight away and dashed out to take the call, feeling enthusiastic and reluctant simultaneously, if that's possible. I wanted to know, but at the same time I didn't really know if I was ready for all of this to be over.

'Did I catch you before you left?' asked Sinéad, the nurse who had been my first point of contact in St Vincent's Ward. I explained that I was in the airport. She gave me the news I suppose I should have been waiting for. They were happy with my scan. There was nothing new lighting up. They'd see me in April. I hung up the phone and went back in to Gordon and the rest of them and I relayed the news with tears in my eyes, still uncertain of how to feel. They seemed happy, but I felt numb, somehow, and was hit with a bout of familial claustrophobia, mumbling an excuse as I pulled away from the group, dragging my suitcase with me.

> *I relayed the news with tears in my eyes, still uncertain of how to feel. They seemed happy, but I felt numb.*

I felt as if they expected me to be excited and happy, but I wasn't feeling anything. I couldn't sit there while they looked at me, waiting for a reaction, because I wasn't having one. If anything, I was feeling disappointment and shame over not being the happy cancer soldier I was supposed to be. Why wasn't I happy? Maybe it would take a few days to sink in, Gordon suggested. Maybe. Or maybe I'd feel it properly once I saw my consultant?

When we arrived in Portugal, Gordon and I bought a bottle of sparkling wine, just in case I felt like celebrating. We left it in the hotel fridge a week later.

The numb feeling travelled back to Dublin with me and remained through my next hospital appointment, where a member of my consultant's team officially gave me the results. She was a very young doctor, whom I had never met. She seemed nervous and excited as she showed me the words 'Complete remission' on the screen.

'Great,' I said, my face betraying my voice.

'This is a good-news day!' she said eagerly.

'Yeah, I know,' I replied, trying to smile.

The disappointment was written across her face. Why was this person, who was arguably getting the world's best news, not reacting? I did my best to feign a bit of excitement, but still I felt nothing.

I was confused, and frustrated. Surely now was the time I should be getting the pay-off, the feeling of jubilation to counteract the horror of the bad news at the beginning? Instead, I found myself avoiding people, dreading the moment I would have to tell them the good news and pretend to be excited. I had been so open about the bad news and yet I couldn't bring myself to talk about the good.

I think I had grown so used to being a person with cancer

I couldn't really remember how to be a person who didn't have cancer. I was used to treatment, and nurses, and hospital, and being taken care of. I didn't really know how to return to normal life. Having said that, there was no way I could return to the life I'd had, because it didn't exist any more. That in itself was scary. Who was I now? Was I a changed person? How would the new Louise fit into the old Louise's real life?

Also, and this is not something I like admitting, but – hey ho, honesty, etcetera – there were some benefits to being sick. I never had to do anything I didn't want to do. If I felt like taking it easy for a day, I could. If I wanted to eat shite all day long, I could. If I wanted a cup of tea, I could ask someone, and they'd get it for me. Now I don't think I took advantage of this too much while I was sick, but

Going back to real life meant going back to responsibilities, and I had really enjoyed not having to worry about anything other than my treatment. In many ways it had been the most relaxed time of my life.

I *could* have. Going back to real life meant going back to responsibilities, and I had really enjoyed not having to worry about anything other than my treatment. I had *really* enjoyed it. It might sound crazy, but in many ways it had been the most relaxed time of my life.

You see, from childhood, I had had an inflated sense of responsibility. I had to take care of my brother. I had to take care of Dee. I had to make sure no one noticed it was vodka in her glass. I had to make sure I was smiling so that no one guessed things were bad at home. I had to make sure that Granny and Grandad weren't worrying too much. I worried about everything. But when I had cancer, for the first time in my life I felt like I only had to worry about me. Not work, not my friends, not my family. Me. And that was a relief.

The days passed and I knew that I would have to share the news of my all-clear publicly. People had been so kind to me when things were bad, I owed them the good news as well. It just so happened that, eleven days after I received that phone call in the airport, it was the Irish Cancer Society's annual fundraising day, Daffodil Day. My Twitter timeline was filled with photos of daffodils and people sharing stories and memories of their loved ones' experiences with cancer. I was sitting in the nail salon, waiting for my appointment, when I thought, Fuck it. Now's as good a time as any.

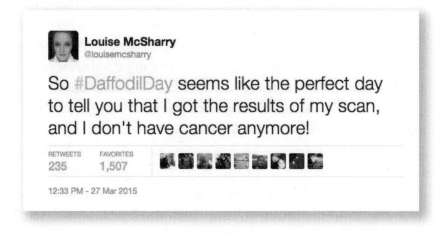

Louise McSharry
@louisemcsharry

So #DaffodilDay seems like the perfect day to tell you that I got the results of my scan, and I don't have cancer anymore!

RETWEETS 235   FAVORITES 1,507

12:33 PM - 27 Mar 2015

I thought my phone was going to melt with faves and retweets. Hundreds of people sent me messages to tell me how delighted they were for me. News articles were written and the commentators were nice. After a while, the joy became contagious, and I started to feel a warmth spread within me. By the time I left the salon, my phone battery was nearly dead and I had sent out the bat signal to my pals. I was ready to celebrate! That night we drank champagne and laughed our heads off. I felt lighter, like I could cope with the idea of moving on for the first time. It was great.

It wasn't a miraculous turnaround, of course. I found it strange to think about the patients I'd seen every two weeks carrying on with their journeys while I was getting back to normal. Tara and Sarah, two friends I'd made during treatment, were still dealing with complications, and it felt unfair that I was able to go back to work and play while they continued the slog of hospital appointments and lived with the uncertainty.

However, I did get back to normal, and six months after the appointment in which I had disappointed the young doctor, I found myself in the clinic again for a check-up. *F**k Cancer*, my TV documentary, had gone out a few days before, and I felt very conspicuous as I walked into the waiting room. If people weren't looking at me, I certainly felt like they were, so I was thrilled to see Tara walk in with her parents. I wasn't thrilled, however, to hear that things had continued to be difficult and complicated for her, and she was looking at another year of treatment. 'She hasn't been as lucky as you,' her mother said, before asking me about my recent wedding.

Not long after Tara arrived, our friend Sarah came in. She had had an awful time of it, having had a lengthy bout of chemo, a big surgery and a course of radiation. She was in the clinic that day to get her results. She was her usual bubbly self, but I could see in her mother's eyes how anxious they were. Sarah was eighteen and had just started nursing college, and she was ready to move on with her life. All they wanted was the all-clear.

My appointment was over quickly. My bloods looked good,

and everything seemed to be in order. 'See you in three months!' the consultant said. 'Give Sarah the all-clear!' I wanted to reply. I felt guilty as I told the gang in the waiting room that everything was turning out well for me. It felt so unfair that I had spent the preceding weeks all over the telly and newspapers, talking about life moving on, when they were still in the throes of it. I said my goodbyes, asking them to let me know how they got on as soon as they could, and walked away, feeling mixed up.

The questions are probably the same for every person who has a life-threatening illness and survives. Why me? Why was my experience so simple when theirs was so complicated? Why have I been so lucky? I struggled with these issues a lot during treatment, and they're still things I think about today. However, you have to get on with it. No one knows why – that's the thing about illness. It can seem totally arbitrary, and totally unfair.

Thankfully, Tara and Sarah both got good news that day. The cancerous activity going on in Tara's body had reduced significantly for the first time in nine months, and Sarah got the all-clear. When I heard the message about Sarah, I felt all of the feelings I had expected to feel the day I had that phone call in the airport. Tears filled my eyes, and I felt a rare kind of delight and gratitude. Maybe you just can't feel that way for yourself. Anyway, I'm glad I got to experience it at last. And now we can move on.

That doesn't mean it goes away, though. In fact, I think it always stays with you. A few times a week something happens that makes me check myself and wonder if I'm experiencing symptoms. I've been tired . . . is that normal tired or cancer tired? I was sweating this morning . . . is that normal sweat or cancer sweat? In those moments I sit still and listen to my body for a moment. I'm okay. I'm okay. It's hard not to wonder if it'll always be that way. It could happen again. What if I'm not okay someday? Will I ever stop wondering? Probably not.

Twenty-one helpful things to do
for a friend who has cancer[*]

1. *Listen*
   Make sure your friend knows they can talk to you about what they're going through. Even the uncomfortable stuff. Avoid rolling your eyes à la Hermione.

2. *Bring them juicy gossip*
   Distraction is invaluable during a long illness, and everybody loves a good piece of gossip. If you're stuck in your house or in hospital, any glimpse into the outside world is a delight.

3. *Buy them a magazine subscription*
   Magazines are great for flicking through when your energy levels are low, or while receiving chemotherapy.

4. *Bring them flowers*
   It's a cliché to get a sick person flowers, but if you're stuck at home for ages anything that brightens up the place is gratefully received. Having said that, if your friend is dealing with severe nausea, it might be better to give the flowers a miss, as the scent may be too much for them.

5. *Offer to do a household chore*
   Nobody ever likes cleaning the bathroom, but if you're spending a large portion of your time laid up in bed, jobs like that certainly aren't what you want to do when

* First published on BuzzFeed, March 2015

you feel well enough to get up and out. A dirty house can be a harsh reminder of a sick person's limitations, so this would be much appreciated.

6. ***Give them some fancy body cream***
Smellies may usually be a bit of a boring present, but chemotherapy can ravage the skin, leaving it dry and occasionally reptilian. A good body cream will be appreciated, although be careful of anything that's heavily scented unless you know that your pal isn't suffering from nausea.

7. ***Let them play with your Tinder***
Truth be told, this is something nice you can do for any of your friends who aren't Tindering themselves. Flicking through the profiles when it's not your romantic life at stake is a genuine thrill.

8. ***Give them a really nice lip balm***
When your body is run down your lips often become dry and sore, so a really nice lip balm is essential. This goes for guys, too. Sore lips are sore lips, no matter what your gender!

9. ***Get them a Netflix subscription***
Don't forget to add some recommendations, too!

10. ***Treat them to a visit from your pet***
Can you think of anything more uplifting than a cuddle with a cute puppy or kitten? If you have one at your disposal, share the wealth. Consider your pet's temperament,

of course, and check first, but if your friend is up for it this could be just what they need.

11. *Do their supermarket shop for them*
Or, the next time you visit, just bring along some basics they can keep in the cupboard.

12. *Offer them lifts*
Your friend will almost certainly need help getting to and from the hospital for treatment and appointments. Even those who drive may not feel well enough after a day of chemo. A lift is an easy way to offer significant help.

13. *Use the post*
A nice card or letter through your letterbox can give even the grimmest days a bit of a lift.

14. *Treat them to a night in a spa hotel*
Your pal probably won't be allowed to travel much during treatment, so a night at a nearby spa hotel can feel like an incredible escape. Keep an eye on sites offering deals to avoid breaking the bank and be sure to check ahead which treatments are and aren't suitable for people with cancer.

15. *Cook them a delicious meal*
There will probably be days when your friend barely has the energy to get out of bed, let alone prepare themselves a dinner. Nutrition is important during cancer, so having a couple of meals in the freezer for days like that can be a massive help. Check in with your

friend ahead of time to make sure that their freezer isn't too full, and that there aren't any foods they've suddenly gone off during their treatment.

16. Send them a big list of recommendations

Your friend will probably have a lot more time to read, watch and listen than they're used to, so will exhaust their 'to watch/read/listen' list pretty quickly. Put together a document full of books, films and podcasts you think they'd like but may not already be clued into. They'll love you for it.

17. Give or lend them an e-reader

Lugging a heavy bag to and from chemo is annoying, but entertainment is essential. Lighten your friend's load with an e-reader filled with books you think they'll enjoy. Try to include some light and frothy stuff, too. On tough days, their brain might not be able for anything too hefty.

18. Bake them something with ginger

Ginger is a great natural remedy for nausea so, if you know your friend is suffering, get baking. (Or buying. Buying is also acceptable.)

19. Don't take it personally if you don't see or hear from them

If your friend cancels plans, or doesn't pick up the phone, it's almost certainly not about you. Low energy levels and unexpected sickness often prohibit someone with cancer from doing the fun things they had planned to do. Also, if they're lucky enough to have lots of friends and family, then their phone probably never stops ringing. Sometimes, they just won't be up for the chats. Sometimes, they won't be up for anything.

20. Ask them what they need

Sometimes, it's difficult for a person who's normally independent and self-sufficient to ask for help, so don't be offended if they say they don't need anything, but don't necessarily believe them either. Be persistent, and offer some of the specifics on this list if they keep turning you down. However, also keep in mind that, sometimes, what they need is space.

21. Keep in mind that needs change

Cancer and its treatment can go on for a while, and what someone needs at the start can be different to what they need at the end. Don't assume, if your mate said they were fine at the start, that they're fine six months in. Cancer treatment is tough and may make your friend feel worse and worse as it goes along, despite the long-term positive outcome. Keep checking in.

5
Fat

'Fat, fat, fat, fat, fat, fat!'

Here is what it has been like for me to be a fat woman with no body confidence. I have spent the majority of most days over the last thirty-three years thinking around twenty to thirty times a day that I am a disgusting, lazy failure. Every time I see another woman I subconsciously assess whether or not I am bigger or smaller than her, and most of the time I am bigger, so I feel like shit. When I am with a thin woman I spend ages trying to figure out if she is naturally thin (better than me), or if she works hard at it (better than me). I pore through magazines, looking at clothes I can't wear because the women in the magazines are better than me and are not slobs. When I'm sharing a seat with someone on a bus or a train, I press myself to the window or sit on the very edge of the seat, for fear that I take up too much space. If I somehow find the balls to go swimming, I cover myself with a T-shirt and make sure to jump into the pool as quickly as I possibly can so that the people around me don't have to gaze at my obscene flesh for too long.

I have spent hundreds, if not thousands, of euro on clothes I will never wear, due to living in the false belief that, someday, the diet will work. Someday, the thin Louise will get out. Someday, I will be better. This expenditure results in having a wardrobe full of clothes, none of which fit me and all of which serve only as a reminder that I am revolting, and lack self-control and, frankly, don't deserve to wear nice things.

For years I avoided going shopping with friends, claiming to hate it, when in fact I would have loved to shop but I knew the shops they went to had nothing for me. I have lied to avoid countless activities over the years because I was afraid I was too fat for them. Sun holidays. Horse riding. Sea kayaking. Hiking. Swimming. Going on a boat. Sitting in the middle seat of a car.

> *I have lied to avoid countless activities over the years because I was afraid I was too fat for them. Sun holidays. Horse riding. Sea kayaking. Hiking. Swimming. Going on a boat. Sitting in the middle seat of a car.*

Apart from the ways I have tormented myself internally, I have spent much of my life convinced that thin people are judging me. If I'm eating in public, then every thin person around me must be wondering why I'm eating when food is the last thing I need. On the occasions I have ventured into a gym I have been certain that all the fit, thin people in the place are secretly laughing at me. For many years I felt guilty any time a normal-sized person had to hug my horrible fleshy body. I would recoil and pull away as early as possible so they didn't have to be in contact with my fatness any longer than was absolutely necessary.

It's really no surprise that I spent so many years feeling this way, while for most of that time my body was average-woman-sized or smaller. We live in a world that is absolutely sizeist. In childhood, we learn that 'fat' is one of the worst things we can call another person. Worse for most little girls than 'mean', 'dishonest' or 'stupid'.

I can't ever remember a time when I wasn't aware of being overweight. I'm not saying that all of my memories are dominated by an awareness of being fat – though many of them are – but when I reach back into the recesses of my mind to find my first thoughts along these lines, I have to go fairly far back.

I'm no older than five and I'm standing on my front doorstep with my friends from our housing estate. It's summertime, no one has school and the sun is shining. Someone has been to the shop, and they have sweets, but I know I'm not supposed to eat any. I'm not supposed to eat any because I'm on a diet. I'm five, and I'm on a diet. I have to repeat that now, because it is so shocking to me that it was deemed appropriate for that to happen.

I can't remember the exact circumstances around it, but what I recall is our family doctor being involved, and that there was a conversation about my weight and it took place in front of me. It is possible there was an assumption that I wouldn't understand but since I was reading Roald Dahl novels on my own by then, such an assumption would have been wrong.

One way or the other, I was five, and I thought I was fat, and I have thought that ever since. A lot of the time, I've been correct, but some of the time I haven't. That's what's so toxic about calling someone fat. Once you've had the thought that you're fat, the chances are it will stay with you for ever, whether you are or not. In a society in which fat is considered one of the worst things you can be, it's a difficult line of thought to cope with. I would say it has been the number-one challenge of my life. Not my family situation. Not the cancer. Not actually *being* fat either, because the fat itself has presented me with very few challenges. The *thought* of being fat, however, and all the negative associations that come with it in the world we live in, has been torture.

The reality of the situation is that I wasn't really, properly, fat until I was a teenager. When I look at photos of the five-year-old who was on a diet it's clear to me that I was hanging on to some childhood chub, but nothing abnormal. People told me I was pretty all the time, and I believed them. Hadn't I been on the cover of a magazine? 'Precious,' was my well-rehearsed answer to the question, 'What are you?' and I meant it, too. I felt loved and precious. That all fell apart when Dee fell apart.

Ruaidhrí and Ger were not expert in the world of little girls. Ger and I fought every day as she brushed my hair, and the days of neat plaits were gone. Instead, after one particularly bad screaming match, my long hair was cut off. Ger and Ruaidhrí struggled financially, which is understandable since they were only in their twenties and starting their careers as a teacher and businessman. Expensive clothes for us kids were out of the question. The days of pretty, immaculate Louise were over, and cobbled-together, we're-doing-the-best-we-can Louise took her place.

I wish I could say that these superficial matters didn't have an effect on me, but they did. My confidence suffered, and I stood out for all the wrong reasons. I didn't have the right clothes or the right hair. My packed lunch was all wrong. I lived in the wrong part of town. Even my accent became a source of pain. I made painful attempts to conform, but to no avail. I started getting slagged off in school and, along with the slagging, came the dreaded 'You're fat!' It wasn't long before I really was fat.

I'm not quite sure how it happened. I've spent a lot of time wondering about my relationship with food and whether it was affected by going from a situation where it was readily available to one where it was scarce. Or if my parents' rule that we had to ask before we ate something meant that, once I was able to get food for myself, I went for it in spades. I wondered if my love of eating was linked to psychological trauma. And then I wondered if it was just that I really bloody liked food, just like lots of people of all different shapes and sizes, some of whom are able to eat whatever they want, apparently without consequences, and some who aren't. Just bad luck. I no longer really care about the why or the how, but for years I did.

My fatness was the root of everything that was wrong in my life, as far as I was concerned, but I did my best to pretend it wasn't even an issue. I think a lot of fat people do their best never, ever to speak about their feelings about their body, somewhere deep down hoping that the people around them won't notice they're large. On some level, I certainly did, even though people were pointing it out to me at every opportunity.

> **My fatness was the root of everything that was wrong in my life, as far as I was concerned, but I did my best to pretend it wasn't even an issue.**

At the bus stop every morning, two boys spent their time pelting me with crab apples and shouting, '*Fat, fat, fat, fat, fat, fat!*' at me. I never said a thing to anyone about it. I think I felt I deserved it, for the heinous crime of being overweight. It came to a head one day when they threw chewing gum at me on the bus. When I arrived home with my hair clumped around a wad of pink gum I couldn't think fast enough to make up a story for my mom. I confessed what had been going on and, in a rare moment of rage, she stormed around the corner to confront the boys' parents. They were affronted that she would accuse their angels of misbehaving and made it clear where she could go. I begged her to leave it alone.

The summer before I started high school, I was thirteen and starting to feel grown up. My granny and my aunt took me shopping for clothes while I was visiting Dublin, an activity I had always enjoyed as, the rest of the year, clothes shopping was just a dream. After trying a few shops in town, I noticed them whispering to each other. Change of plan, they said with false cheer. We were going somewhere else!

They took me to Evans. My heart sank as I entered the shop, which at the time was really the only option for women beyond a size sixteen. These days, Evans has some cool stuff and sponsors a great young-designer competition each year. Back then, it was a different story. When I went back to school that year I had a wardrobe of clothes better suited to my mother. I was so jealous of my friends in their American Eagle boot-cut jeans and jumpers, but one trip to the shops taught me that, even if I could have afforded them, they didn't exist in my size. It seemed the world had found another way to make me feel like an outsider.

When I got back to America that year, my friends had started hanging out with boys. The day after I got home we met up with the group of guys my friends knew and went for a wander around the town. I was full of stories about my summer in Ireland and incredibly excited about the prospect of this new social life. Was it finally happening? Was I now going to have boy friends? Or maybe even a boyfriend? As we walked down the main street of the town, I recognized two figures walking towards me and called out to them. It was Dee and her then boyfriend Fred. At that time, I hadn't seen or heard from her in more than six months and, emboldened by the giddiness of the day, I chased after her as she crossed the street (presumably, to avoid me). 'Hey!' I said, a trail of boys and girls behind me. 'Oh,' she said, looking me up and down. 'Well, you've gained weight.'

I'll never forget the pain of that moment. It honestly felt like a dagger to the heart. Through all the neglect and danger, she had never been unkind to me but, on this day, in front of all my friends, she decided to say the cruellest thing she could have said. I walked away from her, crying hysterically. The guys, in fairness to them, were incredibly kind, but the shine was gone from the day. I just wanted to go home. As an adult, of course, I know this exchange had nothing to do with my weight and everything to do with Dee feeling badly about herself and lashing out to make herself feel better. She has admitted that since. But, at the time, the message was clear: my fatness had ruined things once again.

One thing that didn't depend on size, though, was my school bag. In Batavia, Illinois, in 1995, the only school bag worth having was a Jansport. At the time, they cost around $40, which was way beyond my parents' budget and, anyway, didn't I have a perfectly good school bag from middle school? Determined to have *something* right, I cobbled together enough babysitting money to buy myself a copy of a Jansport. It might not have been exactly right, but it was close, in a lovely wine colour with light brown leatherette at the bottom. I was delighted with it, and myself, for once. I managed to have two good days with it. On the third day, a boy in the year above me, who I don't think I had ever spoken to, wrote FAT GIRL in giant black letters in permanent marker on the bottom of my bag. I

wept in the toilet as I covered the writing in yet more permanent marker, and lied to my friends about what had
happened later in the day.

People seemed to want to point out that I was fat at every
opportunity, but I couldn't possibly talk about these inci-
dents, such was the intensity of my shame. So, instead, I lived
with it on my own.

When you're fat, the remarks don't stop when school days
are over. Lots of people feel entitled to comment on other
people's bodies and, for years, I just put up with it, too
ashamed to say anything. That was a mistake.

The first time I responded to someone was in the smoking area of The George, one of Dublin's most iconic gay
bars. I was with my friend John, and we were having a drink
and a chat when a guy began to make fun of me behind my
back. He was showing off for his friends, gesturing about
my weight. I could see John looking, and I turned and
caught him at it. I couldn't possibly ignore it in front of my
friend, so I confronted him. 'Do you think I don't know
I'm fat? Do you think I don't own a mirror? If you're going
to slag me off, at least come up with something original!'
He quickly backed down and, red-faced, I turned to John.
Nothing had physically changed, but now I felt exposed.
How could I deny my fatness? I carried on as though nothing had happened but, after a couple of minutes, John said,
'I'm sorry, Louise, but how do you even deal with that?
Does that happen a lot?' I told him that it did, and that I was
used to it. I *was* used to it. But that didn't make it any easier.

There was a power in saying, 'Yes, I am fat. I am fat – so bloody what?'

What did make it easier, though, was acknowledging my

fatness out loud. There was a power in saying, 'Yes, I am fat. I am fat – so bloody what?' Even if I didn't entirely believe it, saying the actual words seemed to make them less hurtful. If I say I'm fat myself, then you saying it to me means nothing! From then on, I started saying the words out loud with frequency. It was the start of something.

G'wan, my body!

When I was in fifth year, my friend Sophie went to Weight Watchers. She'd started going when she was sixteen, and she'd lost two stone. She had put back on a little bit of weight, so she wanted to go back to keep on top of it. When she mentioned it, I quizzed her. What was it like? How did it work? Until now, I had never really considered taking action regarding my weight. This seemed like a solution. Maybe I could be a thin person, after all! After asking her a thousand questions, I decided that I would go with her to her meeting. I walked the thirty minutes to the rugby club near her house where it was held and entered the room nervously and excitedly. The plan seemed simple. Every food had a points value, and as long as I stayed under my points value I would lose weight.

At the next meeting I was three pounds lighter. I was hooked. I diligently stuck to my points and exhibited willpower the likes of which I have not seen in myself since. The only time I strayed from the plan was at the weekends, when I went out drinking with my friends. Technically, drinks had points values, but I had decided, in my teenage wisdom, that they wouldn't count for me. And, as it turned out, they didn't, really. Over the next few months I lost two and a half stone.

I was delighted with myself, and with the admiration I was getting. People commented on my weight loss all the time, from relative strangers at parties to my aunt, who nodded approvingly when she saw me, unwittingly confirming that she had disapproved of me. My mother was so impressed by my willpower and the results that she joined Weight Watchers, too, and became a gold member. Unfortunately for me – or at least that's how I felt at the time – I grew complacent. I felt good, and I looked good enough: surely I should be able to go back to being a normal teenager and eat the same things my friends did? It won't come as a surprise to you that the weight came back on, and more besides. The compliments I had received about my weight loss began to ring in my head as insults. Every time I met someone who had been delighted for me, I felt I could see disgust on their face. I had failed. I was a big, fat mess again. But this time it was worse, because I had wasted all my efforts.

Over the next several years I went back to Weight Watchers a few times, with varying degrees of success, never managing to match the positive experience I'd had the first time. Standing on the scales often felt like humiliation and, when the weigh-in didn't go well, other people's success seemed like a slap in the face. More than once I walked away from a meeting feeling so fed up I binged on delicious, forbidden food to comfort myself. As time went on, the successes were fewer and farther between. I had managed to get myself from a size twenty/twenty-two to a size eighteen by the time I met Gordon when I was twenty-six. The thing is, it's a lot easier to lose or maintain weight when you're single so, once I was happily ensconced in a relationship, the weight came back on. Not a huge amount, but enough to get me back into that 'I'm a disgusting failure' frame of mind. At least some of the time.

Not all of the time, though. At this stage I'd started to question the idea that I was a bad person because I was fat. It had started to occur to me that there were worse things I could be. I'd started to rebel against the narrative, and to go swimming if I wanted to or take a risk and get in a sea kayak.

However, when I got sick in 2014, I became desperate. After feeling rubbish for several months, I convinced myself that it must be my terrible fatness that had me feeling wretched and signed up with a very nice, very expensive personal trainer. I banished carbs from my diet and trained for an hour three times a week. I absolutely hated it. I remember one day crying as I fought to continue moving, and another day having to leave because I started vomiting. People kept saying to me, 'Do you feel great, though?' I didn't. But the weight fell off me.

Again, I got the compliments. So many of them. This time, though, I started to resent them. Why was my weight even of interest to other people? Why was it any of their business?

I was seeing a doctor every week, trying to get to the bottom of my illness. 'You need to stop losing weight,' he said. I couldn't believe it. For years and years I'd been avoiding doctors because of the inevitable scolding I'd receive at each appointment over my weight. Frequently, they'd link whatever small complaint I had to the number on the scales. Now, when I was doing the right things and losing weight, a doctor was telling me to stop?

I couldn't believe that, somehow, I had managed to become the person I had always dreamed of being – a person who could take or leave food. However, I was losing weight because I was dying.

The juxtaposition of the weight loss and receiving my diagnosis was powerful. I was thinner than I had been for years and free of thinking about food. I had no desire to eat and, therefore, I wasn't obsessing over whether I was eating 'good' food or

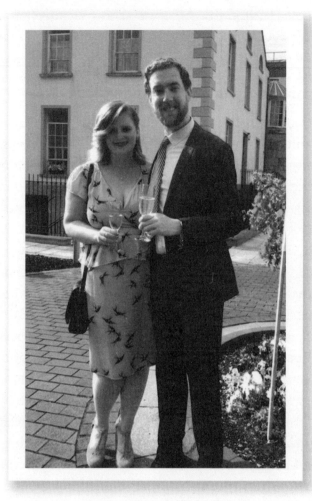

Summer 2014. I was lighter than I'd
ever been, but only because I was dying.

'bad' food. It was incredibly liberating. Every day Gordon quizzed me on what I'd eaten and I got a thrill out of telling him about the tiny amounts of food I'd consumed, ignoring the fact that he was getting more and more annoyed with me. I couldn't believe that, somehow, I had managed to become the person I had always dreamed of being – a person who could take or leave food. A person who didn't have to worry about their weight.

However, I was on a road to death. I had stage-three cancer. I was losing weight because I was dying.

And still the compliments came.

Without intervention, I would certainly have died. Intervention came, though, and when I started getting life-saving chemo, my appetite came back. As a result, I gained weight. Every time I went for treatment I was weighed in order to help them calibrate my dosage. Every session, the number on the scale went up. It really messed with my head.

I knew that it was a good thing that I was gaining weight, because it was an indicator of my body getting back to normal but, at the same time, I didn't *want* my body to get back to normal. I didn't want that gross, fat body.

I won't lie: there were days when I genuinely wished I could go back to the days pre-treatment when my body was, literally, wasting away. Yes, I had a life-threatening illness but at least I was on the road away from fat.

In order to try to compensate for my improving health and resulting weight gain, I did my best to eat very little during the day while Gordon was out. I obsessed over food, one day to the extent that it was pretty much all I could think of, and by the time Gordon got home from work I had worked myself up into a tearful frenzy. I felt like I was losing my mind. Logically, I knew that it was crazy to worry about my weight when my focus should be on getting better, but the high of losing all the weight was still in my mind. If I went back to being properly fat, then everyone who had complimented and congratulated me would be disappointed. *I* would be disappointed. I would be the pathetic mess I had always seen myself as.

After that particularly bad day of hysterics, I knew that

something had to change. I knew it wasn't right to sit on the couch all day staring at a punnet of grapes and a packet of ham. I had to stop. I wasn't really sure how to get away from my obsession, but I knew that, as a general rule in my life, the more I spoke about things, the easier they became. So I started talking. I tweeted about it. I wrote a column about it. I chatted about it with friends. The more I expressed my feelings out loud, the more insane they sounded. I found myself enjoying food again and, while I struggled with the weight gain, my inner voice coached me through it. 'This is not what's important, Louise. *This is not what's important!*'

Once I'd decided that my weight was not what was import-ant in the context of my life-threatening illness, I began to question whether or not it was important at all. If it wasn't worth stressing about during this physically difficult time, then was it worth stressing about ever? Out-side of cruel comments from strangers and the way I beat myself up over it, what negative effect did being fat have on my life? Was it preventing me from doing any-thing, or was I myself preventing myself from doing things and using it as an excuse?

Once I'd decided that my weight was not what was important in the context of my life-threatening illness, I began to question whether or not it was important at all.

When I really thought about it, I realized there were very few things being a fat person stopped me doing. In fact, there were only two things I could think of. The first was high-level physical activity. With walking being my primary method of transportation, I was relatively fit. I mean, I wasn't going to be running any marathons any time soon, but neither were most thin people I knew. Physically, I was just as able as most of my thin friends, and more able than some. Indeed, if I wanted to run a marathon, I was fairly sure I could do, if I put the work in. I thought of the people I'd watched cross the finish line at the Dublin Marathon. They had been all shapes and sizes. I had marvelled at many of them, thinking, *If they can do that, then I probably could, too.* The thing is: I don't want to be an athlete so, really, that point is moot.

The second thing my fatness was stopping me from doing was shopping like thin people do. That's beyond my control. Until the fashion world decides to make clothing for the average woman, I'll have to find my clothes in a limited number of places. That one annoys me because I want to be able to have the same range of options as thin people, and I want to be able to shop in actual shops, instead of having to buy everything online. I want to be able to go shopping with friends and take part, rather than acting as a chaperone.

In many ways, things are improving for plus-size shoppers, but it's still aggravating. But was that reason enough to spend my life rebelling against my body's natural size? Was fashion a good enough reason to torture myself day in and day out about every single thing I ate? Was the impossibility of shopping like thin people a good enough reason to look at myself in the mirror and hate what I saw? To think of myself as a failure whatever my life's successes? I decided that I didn't think it was.

As I continued my journey through chemo, my body got larger but my thinking got better. Instead of focusing on my size, I began to think about all the wonderful things my body was doing for me. As I sat with people during treatment I saw the ways they were struggling and realized I was having a relatively easy ride, and that was all down to my strong body. Though my immune system was compromised, I only ever got one small infection. I had to be hospitalized just once, for three nights – an impressive performance by my body. My bloods were improving. *G'wan, my body!* And, in the end, I didn't have cancer any more, thanks to the chemo and – you guessed it – my body.

Cancer taught me about my body's purpose. I had spent my entire life taking my body's abilities entirely for granted. I had focused on what it couldn't do and what it wasn't. I wasn't a natural athlete. I didn't wear the right-sized jeans. My body didn't look the way I thought it was supposed to. The thing is, my body was built for more than wearing clothes and doing gymnastics. My body was built to keep me going. To walk. To breathe. To keep my heart beating. To keep me alive. How could I continue cursing my body when it was serving its purpose brilliantly?

How could I continue cursing my body when it was serving its purpose brilliantly?

When it had fought off a life-threatening illness for months on end before I was diagnosed, so well that not only was I still working but I was walking to work?

My body is not for show. My body is not to put clothes on. My body is built for a purpose and, until it fails me on that front, I refuse to view it as my enemy.

I am fat

Deciding you don't want to hate your body any more doesn't mean you stop seeing it as the enemy and something to be punished. So I still have bad days. However, I have found that there are ways to counteract the dark thoughts.

For a start, I've started to call myself fat. For a long time, 'fat' seemed like the worst thing anyone could call me, but once I started owning it the word lost a lot of its power. I am fat, and I'm okay with it. In fact, I find it more offensive now when people try to deny my fatness than if they refer to me as fat in the first place. If you're a fat person, you know what I'm talking about.

I find it more offensive now when people try to deny my fatness than if they refer to me as fat in the first place.

You: 'As a fat person, I . . .'
Person: 'You're not fat! Don't say that about yourself!'

The thing is, when you, as a thin person, are horrified at the idea of me – a fat person – calling myself fat, by implication you are saying that you are horrified by me. Already, there are massive industries built on the idea that being a fat woman like me is the worst thing imaginable. Why else do people spend thousands of euros on diet books, diet clubs and liposuction? The message is clear. No one wants to be fat. No one wants to be like me.

I don't really want to hear that message, so I'm choosing not to surround myself with things that reinforce it.

I don't buy magazines any more. I don't look at pictures of women I'm never going to be like because, what's the point? I'm never going to be thin, and accepting this has been glorious.

I refuse to put more importance on weight and size than is necessary.

I no longer comment on other people's bodies, because I know that, while it feels great to get a compliment when you lose weight, you hear them all ringing in your head when you gain it back, and feel like a colossal failure.

I refuse to talk about being 'good' and being 'bad' when it comes to food.

I am not going to accept that part of being a woman is being in constant anguish about your body.

I am not going to accept that part of being a woman is being in constant anguish about your body.

I am not willing to have big chats about weight loss any more. I despise the way that diet and exercise chat appear to have become a conversational fallback for many women, as football is for many men.

I have chosen not to measure success by size any more.

Instead of taking part in the 'nothing tastes as good as skinny feels' dialogue, I am instead working hard to build a world around me that supports my existence. This is relatively easy to do and can have an enormous impact.

The biggest gift we have in this regard are plus-size bloggers. There are now hundreds of women on the internet who are unabashedly living their lives as fat women and refusing to apologize for it. Seeing them looking happy and confident and wearing – SHOCK! – cool clothes, made me realize I could be like that, too.

On my bad days, I think of gorgeous photos I've seen of plus-size women and it gives me a lift. On really bad days – when I can't seem to get through the dark thoughts – I decide to fake it till I make it and emulate one of these women, who have become sort of heroines of mine.

The purpose of many of these blogs is to point other plus-size women in the direction of cool clothes, which has been a godsend. It's saved me traipsing around the shops, trying on the biggest size they have and hoping it will fit. Generally, this resulted in a hefty dose of self-loathing when the largest size didn't work on my body and resulted in me buying whatever I could get on, whether I liked it or not. This is how a lot of plus-size women shop, and there are few things more demoralizing. I have wept more than once in the cruel fluorescent lighting of a fitting room, cursing my lack of willpower and inability just not to eat. There's nothing like blushing while giving the clothes back to the shop attendant, certain they know that the clothes don't fit you and sure that, after you went into the fitting room with them, they rolled their eyes and mocked your size to their colleague. Those days are gone for me, though, because now I have choices (albeit not as many as I would like), and the plus-size blogging community introduces me to more and more choices every day.

The bloggers have also taught me about body positivity and made me realize that most of my self-hatred is based not on real feeling but on a culture which has decided that there is only one type of body which is acceptable – a thin, white one. I've never seen the central message of body positivity put better than it has been by my friend Bethany Rutter on her blog archedeyebrow.com:

> As I perceive it, body positivity does not mean you are posi-tive about your body, or positive about some bodies, or positive about the fact you have a body and aren't a disem-bodied voice floating in the ether. It means radically repositioning how and what we think about which bodies are good and important and valid and worthy of praise. It means doing more than reinforcing the worth and validity of white, thin, cisgender,* non-disabled bodies with no body hair or scars. It means reinforcing the worth of bodies that do not look or function like that, and refusing to strive for goals that necessarily privilege those categories, and more categories on top of those.

In short, we have to try to change the perspective that only one type of body is beautiful. And no, liking our own body is not really enough, but it's a very good place to start.

Body positivity has been having a bit of a media moment, which means that lots of brands and celebrities are getting onboard. Marc Jacobs sent Beth Ditto down the runway; a billboard of plus-sized women went up in Times Square; and Khloé Kardashian posted a photo of plus-size stunner Ashley Graham on her Instagram. Great, right? Well, it kind of is. Yet Beth Ditto can't buy anything from Marc Jacobs, and the women on that Times Square billboard rep-resent only the smallest of plus-size women, and Khloé

---

* Cisgender means your gender self-identity is in alignment with the sex you were assigned at birth.

goes to the gym every single day to maintain her substantial weight loss (while still bemoaning her body issues). It's good to be talking about body positivity, but it's possible that we're missing the point.

Last year the unbelievably beautiful – and thin – model Gigi Hadid made a public statement about body shaming. Online trolls, or 'fat-shamers', as one newspaper called them, had been complaining about her walking the world's runways during fashion week with her big hips and thighs. What they meant is that her body has a shape, rather than being like a walking pipe-cleaner of the type we're used to seeing on the catwalk. In her statement she said she knew she didn't have the same body type as other models but she was just doing her job to the best of her ability. And, anyway, she was fitting into sample sizes.

I found the whole thing depressing. First, that the abuse had become so intense Gigi Hadid felt the need to speak out is horrendous. Second, that the abuse she received was deemed 'fat-shaming' at all. Third, that she felt the need to qualify her argument by telling people she was fitting into sample sizes. The message many fat people will have received from this is 'I don't have anything to apologize for because I'm thin enough to fit into sample sizes but of course if I couldn't, then it would be a different story.'

Gigi Hadid was speaking about her ability to do a specific job – modelling for high-end designers – but when taken in a broader context it seems like yet another thin woman setting the rules of what's acceptable and what is unacceptable.

When people like Gigi Hadid and Demi Lovato are anointing themselves the queens of body positivity, it's no wonder that women who are size tens are consumed with guilt over eating too many biscuits with their tea.

Demi Lovato has done solid work talking about her struggle with an eating disorder and encouraging fans to love themselves, which is great. But she also frequently talks about unapologetically showing off her body because she's 'worked hard to get it'. The implication is clear: you can only show off your body if it's a certain type, the type you have to work hard to get.

It's great to talk about body positivity but, if it's only serving to create a new club of women that excludes other women, it's pointless.

It's also great that more clothing brands are expanding their lines to include bigger sizes, but the way many of them are doing it is questionable. A brand may go to a size twenty-eight ('cos if you're above a size twenty-eight you don't deserve to wear nice clothes?) but is the model they're using a twenty-eight? No.

I recently learned of a company that was adding a 'curvy' range to its line. The clothes started at a size eighteen, but the size-eighteen model suggested for the campaign was deemed 'too fat'. They went with a size-fourteen model instead. So they had to make sample sizes smaller than the actual range for her to wear in the photographs. The women they were selling the clothes to could never look like the model wearing them in the picture. The company was selling a lie and sending out the message that fat women are too unattractive to be looked at. However, we do have money in our wallets, so they'll let us buy their stuff.

Even when companies use a model who is the smallest size in the range, she is almost certainly a beautiful white woman with a perfectly flat stomach and a body with the same proportions as a thin model. She will be held up as a 'curvy beauty' and embraced by the straight-lined small-sized world. She looks like us, they seem to think; she's acceptable. So there's one more way you're failing if you're a fat woman: not only are you fat but, if you have to be fat, you're *the wrong kind of fat*.

There's a reason that a lot of the online plus-size community has started cheering any time a model with a visible tummy is used. It's because we have visible tummies! And maybe we shouldn't have to hide them! Maybe we don't mind them! Maybe we've decided not to be shamed into wearing black sacks disguised as tunics and 'flattering' peplum tops which hide our hideousness!

> *There's a reason that a lot of the plus-size community has started cheering any time a model with a visible tummy is used. It's because we have visible tummies! And maybe we shouldn't have to hide them!*

You see, that's fat-shaming. Fat-shaming is implying, with the way a 'flattering' plus-size clothing range is presented, that you need to hide your gross, fat bits away. Fat-shaming is making the fat girl the butt of the joke in every scene of the movie. Fat-shaming is complaining about how fat you are to a person who is much fatter than you. Fat-shaming is complaining about the fat guy you had to sit beside on the plane. Fat-shaming is talking about bikini-bodies and implying that only certain types of bodies are good enough to wear bikinis.

Fat-shaming is also the obvious things, like the YouTuber who became world famous for saying that fat people smell like sausage and then called it satire.

The results of fat-shaming include being afraid to go to the doctor because, every time you go, he or she attributes whatever you are worried about to your weight. That way serious illnesses get missed.

Fat-shaming also leads to depression, eating disorders and dangerous levels of stress. Above all, psychologists say, fat-shaming frequently leads to increased levels of eating. So, for those people who claim they are trying to help people control their weight when they fat-shame, it has the exact opposite result. Fat-shaming leads to fat gain. Give it up.

Guys *do* make passes at girls with fat asses

It saddens me that I spent years thinking men would never fancy me because I was fat. It saddens me even more that I have friends who feel this way now. It saddens me because it's bullshit. If you are a fat woman who feels this way, ask yourself this question. Are you not getting dates because you're fat *or* are you not getting dates because you've decided you're not good enough to date because you're fat? I would argue that it's almost certainly the latter.

When my weight used to fluctuate, it never fluctuated too much. It was generally the difference between a size eighteen and a size twenty, a small physical difference, but one that had a huge impact on my frame of mind. When I was an eighteen, I fit into *all* the clothes in my wardrobe. When I was an eighteen, I could shop in more of the 'normal' shops. When I was an eighteen, I considered myself more acceptable. And so, when I was a size twenty, I never had romantic liaisons. But when I was a size eighteen, I had as many as I wanted. The reason was simple: I didn't put myself out there when I was a size twenty. I had decided no one would be interested in me, and that I wasn't good enough to be with a guy (any guy, by the way, even the gross, rude, stupid ones). That was the message I

If you're in the mires of self-hatred over your body, it's hard to believe someone saying that if you 'decide' you're attractive, you'll be attractive, but try it.

was putting out into the world with my attitude and actions and, as a result, I was alone.

I know that, if you're in the mires of self-hatred over your body, it's hard to believe someone saying that if you simply 'decide' you're attractive, you'll be attractive, but try it.

There will be some guys who won't be into you, just as there are some guys who aren't into blondes. But that isn't about you not being good enough. It's about them.

Whatever they might feel deep down, fat-shaming results in people growing up thinking it's weird to find a fat person attractive. This especially affects teenage boys, who are keen to fall in line with what's seen as appropriate by their pack. The thing is, the idea that fat people are unattractive is a total lie. Sure, some people may find me unattractive because I'm fat. But I've had plenty of sex with men who had absolutely no issue with it and I've been attracted to a fair few fat men along the way as well.

Just like some men like small boobs and some like big boobs, it's down to personal taste. The blanket ban on fat people being eligible to be considered attractive is bullshit. Just ask the hundreds of thousands of fat people around the world who are blissfully happy in relationships in which they feel beautiful. Or, indeed, fat women who make a living by letting men look at them naked. Some people may want you to believe it's some sort of freak show, but the demand would indicate that it's a case of men finding fat bodies attractive.

I know some of this may come as a shock, but I've got something else to say: for some people, a person being fat even sweetens the deal.

Fatspiration

Earlier today, when I took a break from writing, I noticed that a women's magazine that I really like posted a photo on Instagram for 'fitspiration'. The woman in the photograph is tiny. She has a six-pack and a thigh gap you could drive a car through. According to her own Instagram bio, fitness is her life and, judging by her photos, she is entirely dedicated to it, having it as her full-time job and a personal hobby. She has the kind of body you could only have if fitness was not only your full-time job and a personal hobby but if you also had a natural propensity towards being lean and muscular. Why, then, is it being suggested to the thousands of women who follow this magazine on Instagram that this level of fitness is what they should be aiming for?

The fitspiration hashtag is dangerous. What it says is: 'Look at this person, they are better than you! Why aren't you more like this person?' As women, we spend our whole lives comparing ourselves to other women, wondering why we can't be more like them. It's toxic.

What would you say to a little girl who came home from school upset because another girl was prettier than her? You'd probably tell her she was beautiful but also that looks aren't the most important thing, because she's also smart and funny and good at whatever she's good at. Why do we not give ourselves the same pep talk as adults that we give to children?

Being fat is not the worst thing you can be. I have read too many tragic stories about young women killing themselves with slimming pills, or women whose lives have been destroyed after gastric bypasses left them with debilitating loose skin or other health conditions. It's heartbreaking. I empathize with these women. It is hard to be fat in a world that hates fat people. And we do live in a world that hates fat people.

The hatred and dread of fat people is never clearer than in the responses to the body-positivity movement. Every time a woman writes an article about feeling good about herself while being above-average in size there is a barrage of negative comment. Commentators lament the cost to the health service or claim the writer is 'promoting an unhealthy lifestyle'. Sometimes they just declare that she is 'disgusting'. They seem to be saying that fat people *should* be marginalized and made to feel ashamed. But if fat people aren't ever allowed to be told, 'You look great!' maybe smokers should never be given a compliment either. Or people who eat only junk food but remain thin. Or anyone in a pub having more than the recommended number of units of alcohol.

A 2008 study of lifetime medical costs in the UK found that obese people actually cost the health service less than the 'healthy living'. Sorry, folks! No longer can you blame us fatties for your upset over tax expenditure. It turns out that many fat people are perfectly healthy. As for promoting an unhealthy lifestyle, I fail to see how a fat person writing about the ways they've found to be happy is encouraging other people to become fat. But to argue this point implies that I believe in the motives of those who focus on the health implications of being fat. And I don't believe that most people give a shit about other people's health.

The commentators who find us repulsive are at least honest because the truth is that many people find fat people repulsive. At the root of the negative response to body-positivity among fat people is an inherent distaste for fat people. It's a prejudice like any other. There was a time when being fat was a good thing in the Western world. Now it's a sign of (a) being lower class (because you can only afford, or know no better than to buy, cheap and processed fattening foods) or (b) and worse – if you're middle class, and presumably know enough and could afford to eat 'better' – it's a sign of a lack of self-control. If you find fat people disgusting, then you are prejudiced. And your prejudices will tell you a lot about yourself, your values and your inner fears. Don't try to camouflage your true belief with faux concern about my health and expect me to go back to my fat corner with my tail between my legs.

> *If you find fat people disgusting, then you are prejudiced. And your prejudices will tell you a lot about yourself, your values and your inner fears.*

But what about the fat people who really are unhealthy? I hear you (thin) people ask. What about those whose size negatively affects their mobility or life span? Surely those really fat people shouldn't be encouraged? Surely it's dangerous to pretend that their bodies are okay?

Just stop yourself right there and consider this: *it is none of your fucking business.* If someone's body is a problem for them – in terms of happiness or health – then it's up to them to change it. It's entirely up to them. They do not need your input. In fact, for many people who struggle with their weight, your input only makes things worse.

So, here's my thing. Feel whatever way you feel about your body but think about where those feelings come from. If you hate your body, ask yourself why. Do you hate your body because you are uncomfortable and it stops you doing things? If so, fair enough. However, a lot of the time, I think we hate our bodies because the world is telling us to hate them. The world tells us that fat people aren't as good as thin people and that they are lazy and gluttonous. The world says it's cute if you're a pretty, thin girl who eats 'like a dude'. But if you're a fat woman who eats the same way then it's ugly. The world says that only some people can wear a bikini. The world says that some stomachs are good enough to be on display but other stomachs are not. The world says that some people are attractive and others aren't. The world is full of shit.

If you feel badly about your body because the world says you should, then give the world the finger and find a different way to look at yourself. Look at your abilities. Look at the beautiful things about your body. Be grateful for what it does for you every day. Don't buy into the bullshit.

If you decide you want to lose weight, good for you. It's bloody hard, and I admire anyone who manages to do it healthily and maintain the loss. However, if, for whatever reason, you don't, that's okay, too. You are not less of a person because you are fat. You are not a failure because you are fat. Maybe you just can't lose weight right now because you're going through something difficult and you really need the comfort of beige goods from the deli counter. Maybe you're having too much fun eating out with your pals and enjoying a few drinks at the weekend to give it up. Maybe you're just unwilling to spend any more time stressing about every morsel that goes in your mouth. Perhaps you quite like your body the way it is, though it's not the type the world finds satisfactory.

If, for whatever reason, you are staying fat, then own it. Forgive yourself. Decide that the rest of the world can fuck right off if they think you're going to be miserable just because you're carrying some extra weight.

> **If, for whatever reason, you are staying fat, then own it.**

If you think what I'm saying is easier said than done, try faking it. When you have a negative thought about your body, replace it with a positive one. If you think, 'My fat is squidging over the top of my pyjama bottoms. How gross!' remember that that squidge is exactly what makes your tummy the ideal cat pillow when you lie on the couch. If you find yourself looking at photos of fitness professionals on Instagram and envying their hard, taut bodies, remember that your softness is exactly what makes babies snuggle into you when you hold them. You don't have to hate your body. There is another way.

Even if you decide you want to lose some weight, you still don't have to look at your current state as hideous. You don't have to subscribe to the 'before' and 'after' culture of weight loss. You don't have to look at photos of yourself at your heaviest and think, *Eeew! Gross!* You can lovingly accept yourself for who you were then, and whatever was happening in your life that led to you being like that. Maybe it was that you were in a new relationship and you were spending all your time going for big brunches and drinking bottles of wine on the couch. Or maybe it was a time when you were really depressed and food was a great comfort to you. Either way, you were what you were. You are what you are. And that's okay.

*

I'm heading into another period of weight loss now, and I have mixed feelings about it. In one way, I'm annoyed. I'm annoyed that, just when I've got to a point where I realize my value is not my body's size, I have to get back on the weight-loss wagon. As a result of my cancer treatment, I have fertility issues. In order for me to get IVF – which may be the best course of action if Gor-

> *I'm annoyed that, just when I've got to a point where I realize my value is not my body's size, I have to get back on the weight-loss wagon.*

don and I want to have children – I have to lose a lot of weight. As much as I hate the weight-loss process, I hate it less than I would hate to be told that IVF was the best option for us but that I can't have it because my BMI is too high, and that is the reality for lots of women. So, I have to suck it up and get stuck in.

On the other hand, this time, the script in my head will be different. Other times when I tried to lose weight I felt psychologically better when I was eating 'thin', even if that meant I was going through a dangerous patch of under-eating and calorie-counting. That isn't right. It isn't right to feel virtuous when you're essentially starving yourself and vile when you have a takeaway on a Friday night. It's okay to have a gluttonous weekend from time to time, we shouldn't feel like we're bad people as a result, but that's the reality of the world many of us live in. Our attitude to food and fitness is seriously messed up.

I no longer believe I am 'bad' for eating certain foods and 'good' for eating others. I will not see myself as a failure on days when I don't follow the plan perfectly. I will forgive myself for being a human being who enjoys food and a social life. I will forgive myself for being 'naturally fat', in the same way that people who are 'naturally thin' are forgiven.

How to feel body confident

Buy clothes you *like*!

Fashion rules are bogus, so don't subscribe to the thinking that fat women should only wear a certain type of clothing. For instance, the line about never wearing horizontal stripes is total BS – I wear them all the time. In fact, all of Gordon's favourite outfits of mine are horizontally striped. If you want to wear a shapeless tent because it's comfortable, grand. However, if you want to wear a bodycon dress, that's okay, too. A while ago, crop tops were everywhere, and lots of fat women (and thin women who think they're fat) thought they couldn't wear them. (And Oprah's magazine decreed they shouldn't.) Wrong! Some of my favourite crop-top outfits have been on women who are my size and larger.

The point is to look in the mirror and be happy with what you see. For years, I based that happiness on whether or not my clothes were flattering or hid my fatness, but these days I don't care so much about that. I prefer my outfits to be fun and stylish, even if that means people can tell that I have – shock! horror! – a belly.

> *These days I prefer my outfits to be fun and stylish, even if that means people can tell that I have – shock! horror! – a belly.*

As I have mentioned already (more than once: it's a bugbear of mine!) one of the hardest things about being a plus-size woman is shopping. Though some high street shops extend to a size eighteen these days, most still don't cater for women above a size sixteen. Once the only shops that catered for us were fuddy-duddy shops for older ladies, but now brands have realized that there are fat women under the age of forty-five who want to wear nice clothes. It is possible these days to be fat and fashionable! However, these brands are not sold in shops on Grafton Street or your local high street so you might not know them. Most of them exist solely online, which prohibits fat women from having a true shopping experience, but it is an improvement.

I'm no fashion blogger, but I've been asked lots of times to share some wisdom on where I buy my clothes, so here are some of the websites I like . . .

ASOS

Ask any plus-size woman who's even remotely into fashion and they'll tell you that she couldn't live without ASOS Curve. The brand itself makes on-trend pieces for relatively inexpensive prices, and the site stocks several other fab plus-size brands like super-cool Danish brand Carmakoma and the Manchester-based Alice & You, which nods to vintage styles. Whether you want a pair of jeans or a glamorous gown, you'll have options on ASOS. Yes, it's online, but delivery is usually quick and free and, with the parcel connect service, returns are relatively painless.

Navabi

Navabi is a slightly more upmarket site which is home to several plus-size brands. You'll spend a good bit more here, but the quality will probably be a good bit better, too. If you want to buy a staple piece you'll hold on to for ages, then this is a good place to look.

Boohoo

Boohoo Plus is a relatively new range, and it follows the style of the rest of the site. It offers cheap fashion items, delivered quickly and easily. If you're in your teens or early twenties, this is the place for you, though even auld wans like me might find a thing or two.

Missguided

A little more high-end than Boohoo, Missguided have a plus-size range which is a good place to look if you want something trendy but not too expensive. (You know what I mean. Sometimes you see things you really like but you know that, in three weeks, everyone in the world will be wearing them and you'll be over it, so you don't want to spend much.) Both the Missguided and Boohoo lines are relatively new, so it'll be interesting to see how they develop.

Elvi

I discovered Elvi only recently, and boy am I glad I did. I've always really resented the fact I can't shop in Zara, and I think Elvi will fill that gap for me with its chic, sophisticated items.

Simply Be

Simply Be is a great one-stop shop because it sells absolutely everything in a large range of sizes (fourteen to thirty-two). Because there's so much stuff on the site, you sometimes have to trawl a little but, if you do, you'll find some really stylish gems.

Depop

Another relatively new site which is kind of like what eBay used to be. These days, a huge amount of what's sold on eBay is brand new, but Depop is largely populated by people selling on clothes they don't want any more. Many plus-size bloggers sell their excess clothes here, and once you find and follow them you'll get alerts when items go on sale. You can also filter what you see by size, so you won't have to look at things which aren't an option for you (the ultimate heartbreak!). It's inexpensive and easy, and I'm a big fan of Depop.

eBay

For a long time I ruled out eBay as a place to shop for plus-size clothes but, after noticing some of my favourite bloggers' finds online, I gave it a go and it's definitely worth a look. Search for 'Plus size' and you'll get hundreds of thousands of results, but you can narrow things down by searching specifically for your size or the kind of thing you're looking for. It's a bit of an effort, but worth it sometimes, especially if you find a particular shop or seller who makes things in a style you like. You can make that shop or seller a favourite, and then stay up to date when they post new items.

. . . And here are some good options for high-street shopping:

Evans

The shop that used to be our only option is still going and, while there are still plenty of mumsy items there, it's worth a look. Evans now sponsors an annual design competition which results in some really fashion-forward items becoming available, and they also collaborated with Beth Ditto for a range in 2009. (*Please, Evans, more of this!*)

New Look

New Look's standard range goes to an eighteen, which is better than some high-street shops, and they also have an Inspire range which goes to a size thirty-two in some items. The quality isn't always amazing, but it's a good option for inexpensive items which generally keep up with current trends.

Marks and Spencer

All right, I know, traditionally, this has been a place where your granny shops, but M&S is honestly one of my favourite places to shop in real life. You'd be surprised what you can find if you keep your eyes open, and the quality is usually really good. Most of the nicest stuff only goes up to a size twenty – they'd really want to sort that out!

Dunnes

Same goes for Dunnes, although their standard range goes up to a slightly bigger size. They're not always the trendiest, but they're great for basics. If only they'd expand the lovely Savida range beyond an eighteen! (*You're losing money there, Dunnes!*)

Cos

Although there's just one full shop in Ireland (and a concession at Brown Thomas) this shop has become a lifeline for me. Technically, the range only goes up to a large/eighteen; however, so many of their garments are oversized that I frequently find lovely things to wear here (and so do plus-size pals of mine in my size and larger).

Forever 21

Yes, the plus-size section is frustratingly small in the context of an enormous three-storey shop, but at least it's there. As is the case in the rest of the shop, the clothes are young, trendy and cheap.

The most important thing I've learned when shopping is to ignore the size on the tag. We all know sizes are inconsistent, to say the least, from shop to shop, so if you're a size eighteen but you find that the twenty is too small, don't stress. Don't let it get you down. You may find that, in the next shop, it's the sixteen that fits you. Neither should you be afraid to try things on just because, by number, it's too small for you. If it's stretchy or oversized, you'd be surprised what you can fit into. You may not always be wearing the garment in the style it was imagined but, if it looks good and you're comfortable, what does it matter?

Please don't stop yourself having nice clothes because you're fat. Please don't spend your life saying, 'I'm not buying any more clothes until I lose the weight.' You might lose the weight, you might not, but you deserve to feel good in the interim. You deserve to put on something that makes you feel pretty and nice.

Chub rub is a practical issue which will annoy you if you're fat. Sort it out and you're good to go. Chub rub is the chafing that occurs when the thighs rub together. This is not solely an issue for fat people; lots of slim people with powerful thighs experience it, too. It is exacerbated by sweating so is especially bad in warm weather, precisely the time you want your thighs to be flapping freely in the wind. For some people it's a source of shame. But you need not feel ashamed, and you also need not suffer with the rub.

Over the years, I've tried out lots of different solutions, and here is what I've found. The simplest and most reliable solution is to wear bicycle-style shorts under your skirt or dress. You've probably figured that out if you have this problem. If bicycle shorts are too heavy for the time of year, Evans sell 'comfort shorts' which come in black, nude and white and are made out of a much lighter material, more akin to tights than actual fabric. These are my go-to guys.

Another fabric option you can try is Bandelettes, which are essentially lacy bands you position on your thighs where they come into contact with each other. These are prettier and sexier than shorts but require a bit of trial and error to figure out where the best position is and to get a pair that stay up all day.

However, sometimes you don't want to wear an extra garment at all. Sometimes your dress is too short or you want to feel the breeze on your legs. On these occasions, you essentially have two options. You either make your thighs very, very dry, or very, very greasy. Both of these options create a scenario where your thighs can slip past each other with relative ease. The downside to both is that you have to repeat regularly through the day.

If you're going to go the dry route, your common-or-garden baby powder is a good option. But even better is Lush's dusting powder, which has a longer-lasting effect. The Lush products come in small bottles so are handy to throw into your handbag. If you're going for baby powder, you can get a travel-sized bottle relatively easily.

If you're going to go the greasy route, you have lots of options. Any lubricant will work, to a certain extent, and you'll find specifically formulated chafing gel in most pharmacies. Another option is a little tin of Vaseline, which is easily found and handbag appropriate. Since there are better options, I only use this if I'm stuck.

The best thing, really, is to test out a few methods and figure out what works for you. I suffered through many a summer wearing opaque tights and trousers because I felt like they were my only option, but those days are gone. My thighs are bleedin' delighted to be free!

As you know, I adore make-up and, if you are into it, it's a great way to focus on the positive and celebrate yourself. Here are my current favourite beauty products, and in each case the cheaper option is almost as good, if not as good, as the spendy one. Why ever splurge, then? Because, sometimes, you just want to feel fancy!

Mascara

Save: Maybelline Lash Sensational Mascara (like the YSL below, but doesn't dry out after four weeks)

Splurge: Yves Saint Laurent Faux Cils

Foundation

Save: Bourjois Healthy Mix Serum

Splurge: Yves Saint Laurent Touche Éclat

Brows

Save: Maybelline Brow Drama

Splurge: Laura Mercier Eyebrow Gel

Bronzer/contour

Save: Sleek Contour Kit

Splurge: Charlotte Tilbury Filmstar Bronze & Glow

Red lipstick

Save: Rimmel Kate Moss

Splurge: Charlotte Tilbury Red Carpet Red

Other lipstick

Save: Sleek True Colour

Splurge: Nars Audacious

Liquid eyeliner

Save: L'Oréal Super Liner Superstar

Splurge: Écriture de Chanel

Eyeshadow for blue eyes

Save: Sorry, but there actually is no cheaper version of the Bobbi Brown below, but it's worth it!

Splurge: Bobbi Brown Camel

Eyeshadow palettes

Save: Sleek eyeshadow palettes (loads of colour, loads of pigment, good all round)

Splurge: Charlotte Tilbury's palettes (there's one for everyone, and they're easy to use, even if you feel clueless about make-up, and there's a YouTube video to go with each one!)

Concealer

Save: Rimmel Wake Me Up

Splurge: Kevin Aucoin Sensual Skin Enhancer (this is a dream product which can do lots of different things. It's pricey, but absolutely worth it, because it lasts for ever)

Finally, the other key thing to do to work on your body confidence is to follow women you *admire* who look *like you*!

If you want to be stylish while fat, you have to work harder than your average woman, which is why I adore following loads of fat babes on Instagram so I can be inspired by their successes. Some of my favourites are Danielle Vanier (@daniellevanier), Bethany Rutter (@archedeyebrow), Nicolette Mason (@nicolettemason) and Isabell Decker (@dressingoutsidethebox).

I cannot recommend this highly enough: it's easy to think the only women in the world who are beautiful, stylish and charismatic are the skinny women celebrated in most of the media. Broaden your horizons and you'll discover a world of fabulous fat women who look beautiful, individual and amazing and have lots of interesting things to say about lots of things.

Getting the perfect beach body

Fooled you! You already have the perfect 'beach body' – the one you're in. As you know, my body-confidence problems started early on, so there was never a time I felt comfortable revealing myself to the extent of wearing a bikini. For years, I avoided swimming and sun holidays because I was too ashamed of my body to have it be seen in public. I feel sad when I think about it. I missed out on so many fun trips and activities for such a bullshit reason.

Eventually, I decided I couldn't continue this way and planned a holiday with my friend. While away, I realized that my paranoia about my body only drew attention to it. There were all kinds of bodies on display by the pool. Yes, some of them were gorgeously brown and lithe, but some of them were the kind of bodies which had seen a lot of fun. Maybe they'd had fun in restaurants, or maybe they'd had fun growing children inside them, maybe they'd spent years basking in sunlight. They were not perfect. They were experienced. None of the women with these bodies seemed at all bothered that they were on display, and I found this inspiring. When I went on my next holiday I decided to pretend not to be bothered.

I bought the nicest one-piece swimsuit I could find and went on holiday with Gordon and a group of lads. A group of *lads*! My actual worst nightmare. The voices in my head were going crazy, telling me that Gordon was bound to be ashamed of me and all the other guys would be wondering what he was doing with me. They'd probably find it hard even to look at me because I was so fat and gross.

On the first day, I wore my cover-up until just before lying down on a sun bed and stretching out my body to make my stomach seem as flat as possible. If I wanted to get into the pool, I'd put my cover-up back on *while I was still lying down*. Then I would walk to the side of the pool and only take it off again at the very last moment before jumping into the water as fast as possible so people weren't subjected to the sight of my body for too long. Frankly, it was exhausting and I wasn't really enjoying myself, so on Day 2 I decided to change tack. On Day 2, I was going to fake it. Okay, I wasn't feeling very confident but I would just pretend that I was and maybe everything would be all right.

Would you believe, everything *was* okay? The lads, of course, didn't give me a second glance, and I was able to relax so much more. Yes, I still had the dark thoughts, but I ignored them and told myself that people like me had been wearing swimsuits for years and it really wasn't that big a deal. By the end of the holiday the bad thoughts were fewer and fewer, and by the next holiday they were almost gone.

Don't get me wrong, I still had my moments on holiday. Once, after the holiday with the lads, I was with a group which included some women who had what were 'perfect' bodies in my eyes at that time. I envied them, of course, but I was determined to seem fine with myself at the very least. One of the best days I had on that trip was when Gordon attempted to teach me to dive into the pool, which required me to climb repeatedly out of the pool in my togs and stand beside it, fully on display, while Gordon modelled the correct positioning for me. Was anyone thinking nasty thoughts about my body? I doubt it – because they were far too busy laughing at how ridiculously bad I was at diving. Another activity on that holiday included creating a group synchronized-swimming routine which started with us sliding off the edge of the pool into the water like penguins. Flattering? No. Did I care? No. Because I realized that I had missed out on so much fun, being ashamed of my body. I had sacrificed too much.

Gordon attempted to teach me to dive into the pool. Was anyone thinking nasty thoughts about my body? I doubt it – because they were far too busy laughing at how ridiculously bad I was at diving.

Ahead of my next holiday, in 2015, there was a bit of a movement online. The fatkini had become a topic of conversation and women of all shapes and sizes had started posting photos of themselves online wearing bikinis. So many of them looked fantastic I started to think that maybe I should consider wearing two pieces instead of togs which were tight, not that comfortable and a pain to get on and off every time I went to the loo. I was going to order a bikini online, but they were expensive and the best options were in America (GabiFresh's line for Swimsuits for All), and I was afraid that it might arrive and not be the right size. Then, fortunately, Forever 21 launched a massive range and I bought three!

The bottoms were really high-waisted and the top came down quite low, so it was really only a sliver of skin which would be showing, but it felt like a big departure. I was delighted to have a few swimwear options while I was away. From a practical point of view, it was great to be able to go to the loo without having to wrestle off togs and sit naked on the pot, terrified that someone would bash the door in. And it was fun being able to talk about bikinis! One of the worst things about being fat is being excluded from ordinary conversations with friends. This time, I could join in and I got loads of compliments on my fab gear.

I was so happy I even took a picture of myself in the mirror! A picture! In the mirror! Of myself half naked! I wanted to share it online, to sort of pay it forward – the bikini photos of women of all shapes and sizes I'd seen online had had a huge effect on me, so it seemed only fair to post one

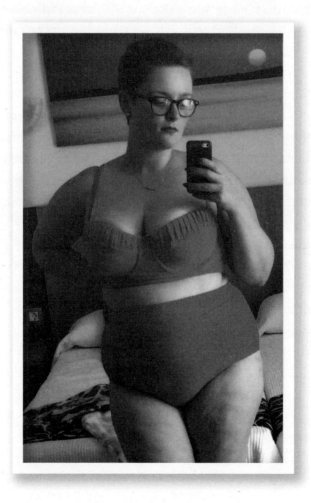

myself. However, I knew that, if I tweeted it or Instagrammed it or put it on my blog, it'd be on various websites within twenty minutes. I was brave, but I wasn't really brave enough for a day of getting Twitter alerts along the lines of '2fm star's brave body baring'.

I still want to share it because I want to encourage you to shake off whatever misconceptions you have about what you are or aren't allowed to do based on your body type. You can do whatever you want. You should do whatever you're comfortable with. I'm hoping the picture reproduced in black and white and buried in the pages of this book will be too hard to reproduce online!

You may not be comfortable enough to wear a bikini today, but maybe if you see a hundred photos of women who look like you over the course of the next year you'll feel comfortable enough to do it next summer. And let me tell you, you will feel amazing. And you will feel silly, because no one will think anything of it. And you will feel like a rock star, because you have overcome a fear and you will realize that so many of the shackles on you are of your own creation.

Fatkinis for ever!

6
Love

Heartbreak

I might as well just say it. Break-ups are probably one of the worst things you ever have to endure as a human being on this earth. No matter which side you're on, if you're a decent person, it's going to be awful. I have been on both sides, and neither is good, but I've only had my heart broken once. My eyes are prickling with tears just thinking about it, which is funny, because I'm now married to the man who broke my heart.

Gordon and I had been together for five months when things started to go a little funny. They had been going really well, and the beauty of our relationship was that it was truly uncomplicated. I would argue that any relationship worth its salt will be uncomplicated at the start. I mean, logistically, we had our problems: I lived in Galway and he lived in Dublin, but we wanted to be together so we made it work. If I texted him, he texted me back. If I said I'd call him, I would. It was simple and straightforward. There was no game-playing. As a result of this, when he seemed out of sorts towards the end of December, I knew something was wrong.

We spent New Year's in Doolin, County Clare, with a gang of friends. It was brilliant in every way, except I had a sense of impending doom. I confided in a pal, who told me to stop being silly. 'You'll ruin this,' she said, having hung out with us a lot over the preceding months. 'He's mad about you.' And he was . . . or he had been. So I tried to chalk down the funny feeling to paranoia. The thing is, I've never really been wrong when it comes to gut feelings with guys. Other times I'd tried to convince myself that things were going well when really they weren't at all and I'd always known the truth on some level. And this time, every fibre of my being was telling me that things weren't right. I tried to ignore it and paste a smile on my face, but when we got back to my apartment in Galway I had to confront the issue.

I was right. Something *was* wrong. An old flame had surfaced, and he needed to figure out his feelings. He was confused and upset. I was confused and upset. We were both crying when he left the apartment to catch his bus back to Dublin. I sat just inside the door for ages, hoping he'd turn back. Hoping he'd arrive at the door telling me he'd made a terrible mistake. He didn't.

I went through the full range of emotions that night, weeping throughout. I felt angry, and hard done by, and sad. The crying continued over the course of the week, during which I got up at 5 a.m. every day to present three hours of happy, sunshiny breakfast radio. We were in touch every day that week, while he tried to figure out what he wanted. It was excruciating and, after having a panic attack in work one day, I called time on it. I remember standing outside my friend's apartment on the phone to him, saying, 'If you still don't know, then that's it. It's done.' He had been honest with me about the whole thing throughout, which I appreciated, but in a way it only made things worse. I had finally – *finally* – found a brilliant, lovely, honest man, and it had gone to shit. Again.

On the Friday of that week I had an appointment to get my

I had finally – finally – found a brilliant, lovely, honest man, and it had gone to shit. Again.

hair done. I was there for five hours. This is not an advice book, but if I was going to give you one piece of advice it would be this: *do not go and sit in a chair in front of a mirror for five hours when you're recently heartbroken.* I wept more or less non-stop while the staff of the salon did their best to make me feel better with jokes and an incredible variety of sweets. I felt guilty, on top of being heartbroken, and when I got on the bus to Dublin afterwards I started crying and didn't stop until I got there. I had taken that bus so many times over the course of our relationship with him in my mind the entire time, so the fact that this time I was going to Dublin to say goodbye to him killed me.

The next day I went to his apartment with freshly done hair, wearing my new red coat as armour. We sat side by side on his couch while I laid down the law. I was going to delete his phone number and unfriend him on Facebook. I would not be emailing him. Please would he not contact me. I explained that it wasn't because I was angry at him, and it wasn't because I didn't care about him, but that if I was going to move on with my life it was what I needed to happen. He seemed to understand. Then I told him that he was brilliant, and I walked out the door.

It was important to me to leave in control of the situation, and I have always encouraged friends in similar situations to do the same. One of the worst things about someone ending a relationship with you is the feeling of turmoil. You find yourself in a situation where you're wishing and hoping for something to happen but that something is entirely in the power of someone else. I really believe a clean break with no

I really believe a clean break with no contact is the only way to go.

contact is the only way to go. People argue with me on this sometimes, citing a desire for friendship, long histories, family involvement, and so on, but – assuming there are no children involved (and that's a quite different scenario) – I really think these are all excuses. The reality is that, if you're in contact, then you are going to be consumed by the person and the situation even more than you already are. You will watch your phone. When it rings, you'll wonder if it's them. You'll wake up each morning and check your phone for a text from them. You'll comb their Facebook page for clues of them moving on. Any interaction with a member of the opposite sex (or the same sex, depending on your preference) will seem like a flirtation. You'll create elaborate tales of their new life with their new romantic partner in your head. You will torture yourself beyond the realms of the unbearable pain you're already experiencing because of the break-up itself.

In a clean-break situation, the worst you can do is obsessively check their Facebook picture every day in case they've changed it and in case there are any indicators of happiness in the background. Because they are not allowed to be happy while you're miserable, that's for sure. And I don't say that sarcastically.

After I issued the no-contact order, I went back to my life in Galway. I put on my happy face and went out every night, always looking for an after-party so I could avoid going home and getting into my bed alone. I listened to Noah and the Whale's *The First Days of Spring* all day, every day (which, by the way, is the ultimate break-up album and happened to come out the week we broke up). I wept in friends' houses until I felt a tolerable weeping period was up, and then I wept alone at home.

After two months it felt ridiculous still to be upset about a relationship which had gone on for only five months, but I tearfully confessed to my best friend that I just couldn't seem to let go of it. I had really thought it was something special. It seemed so bloody unfair that it was over.

Why am I banging on about this so much? Well, because I think it's important that people know they are not alone in their break-up pain. And, also, I think that when we get distance from our own break-ups we forget sometimes just how agonizing they are, and it's probably good to remember the pain so we can give our newly or recently heartbroken friends the kind of support they need.

As it turned out, Gordon and I got back together after two months of no contact and abject misery. The issue that needed to be resolved got resolved and, after consulting with my friend Michelle as to whether or not it would be appropriate, he arrived on my doorstep in Galway to declare his love for me. It was probably one of the best days of my whole life.

Bride fail

I have always wanted to get married. I was never one of those girls who went through a phase of debating whether or not they believed in it or proclaiming that they would never need a piece of paper to legitimize their relationship. Nope, I always knew that marriage was a goal for me. But when I finally got engaged I was a total failure as a bride-to-be.

Though I had always wanted to get married, the wedding was not something I had ever thought about in any detail. When I imagined it, all I would think about was the moment when I would walk down the aisle, looking at the man I was going to marry. When I was in bad relationships, I found myself picturing that moment and filling with dread. In good relationships, I felt a warm glow. It was an excellent barometer of whether or not I should break up with someone. (I think asking yourself who you'd bring with you if you won a holiday is a good indicator, too. If your SO is not the one, then maybe they're not The One.)

Other than that, I never gave the ceremony or reception a single thought. As a result, when Gordon and I got engaged, I didn't really know what to do next. I wasn't sure exactly what kind of wedding I wanted, but that was no big deal because we had *loads* of time to figure it out. Little did I know that, if I wanted to get married in the next eighteen months, I should have started booking things the day after our engagement. At least, that's what it felt like.

Gordon's insistence that I be absolutely blindsided by his proposal meant that we had never chatted about weddings all the time we were going out. And I was so delighted to be engaged to him I intended to savour the feeling and take my time about making plans. In any case, we wanted to figure it all out together.

At first, I enjoyed talking about our engagement. Everyone was really happy for us, and I was basking in the joy of taking the next step towards the life I'd always wanted. But I didn't enjoy the chats for long.

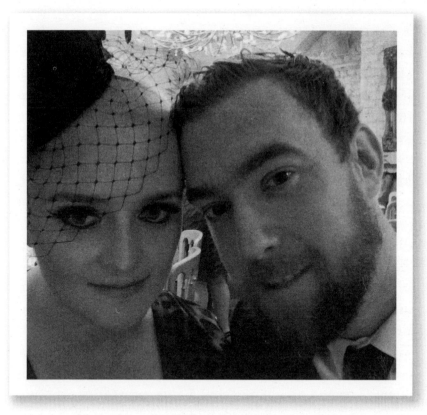

Gordon did most of the work planning our wedding. I found the whole thing really boring.

For one thing people seemed to expect me to be able to tell them exactly what we were planning for our wedding just days after the engagement. They seemed shocked when I said we didn't know and were taking our time. I couldn't believe the pressure people put on us to get things booked. About six weeks after our engagement I was in the pub with a group of women, all of whom I am very fond of, when I found myself being told that if I didn't get shopping for my dress promptly then I probably wouldn't be able to get one. I scoffed and said that was ridiculous, that I could walk into a shop the following day and buy a wedding dress if I wanted to. They looked at me disapprovingly.

Once I was tuned into this new world of being a bride-to-be, I was shocked when I saw people around me getting engaged and booking their reception within the same week. I wondered how they were doing it. Anyone would think they had been planning it long before they got engaged . . . (Spoiler: they had.)

I kept waiting for the interest to come, but it never really did. I got excited about the venue, the music and the food but, once that was all sorted, I really wasn't that bothered. Gordon did most of the organizing of our wedding and I could feel my eyes glazing over every time he started talking about it. For example, when he presented me with prices for the mini-bus service, I just said, 'Yeah, that's grand.' It *was* grand, I really didn't care! Inevitably, we started arguing about it. He was, understandably, frustrated that I wasn't even replying to emails about decisions that needed to be made regarding equipment and invitations, and I kept wondering what was wrong with me that I wasn't interested. I felt guilty about it for the duration. He asked me how he was supposed to feel that I didn't even want to talk about this momentous occasion. I could see where he was coming from but my disinterest wasn't a reflection of how I felt about him or getting married; it was a reflection of how I feel about event planning. I'm not into it. That's probably why I didn't choose it as a career.

At the end of the day, your wedding, aside from the ceremony itself, is a big party. A big party you spend a year and a half or so planning. I don't know about you, but I can't think of any party I would want to talk about endlessly for eighteen months. I found the whole process really boring, and every time someone asked me how the plans were going I struggled to muster up the excited tone I knew they were expecting. I frequently found myself desperate to get away from people whom I genuinely like. It seemed that, once I became an engaged woman, the wedding was all anyone wanted to talk to me about. I could practically see the disappointment on people's faces when I didn't serve up the dose of 'Excited Blushing Bride 2015' they wanted.

I can't think of any party I would want to talk about endlessly for eighteen months. I found the whole process really boring.

(I understand that people need to make small talk and therefore we ask each other banal questions like 'How is work?' or 'How's the love life?' or, when the person is engaged, 'How are the wedding plans?', but I think we could work on our conversation openers. How about 'What's the most delicious thing you've eaten recently?' Or 'What TV show are you bingeing on at the moment?')

Friends of mine got married in this period and many of

them spoke about the blues they experienced afterwards. 'What am I supposed to do now?' they said, mourning the project. I couldn't relate on any level.

After a while, I was sick of feeling guilty and began to question the pressure. Why did I feel like I should be a 'typical bride', one who obsessed over details and relished every second of the planning? Why was it the bride who was supposed to be into all this, anyway – why not the groom? I didn't buy into gender stereotypes in any other area of my life, so why was I allowing myself to feel down because I wasn't playing the traditional role?

The day we went to get our marriage licence the sun was shining in Dublin. I walked to the civil registration office on Lombard Street, listening to the Róisín Ingle podcast. She was talking to the comedians PJ Gallagher and Joanne McNally about their show *Separated at Birth*. As the name indicates, the two of them felt an instant connection when they met, partially because they had both been adopted from towns in Roscommon twenty miles apart.

The conversation was easy between the three of them, and I found myself thinking about the differences and similarities between my adoption and those of people who come to their parents via a more traditional route. Joanne and PJ had both met their birth parents and found the experience rewarding, but Joanne was honest about some of the more difficult elements of forming a relationship with the mother who had given her up at a time in her life she would never be able to recall: 'We're getting on really well . . . It's finding the levels. She said she loved me from the second she opened the letter from me, so for her it's been kind of like an outpouring, it's difficult. We'll get there, it's going to be amazing.'

It was the first time I had heard someone else describe a relationship that was anything like the one I have with my own bio-mom. It's complicated, and difficult to explain, and difficult for me to understand, so it was a big moment when I heard Joanne speaking in a way that was so familiar to me. I found myself listening back to that section of the podcast over and over again. I sent Joanne a DM on Twitter as I walked towards our appointment to make our forthcoming wedding official. When I arrived, I was excited. I took a photo of the civil registry office sign and forced Gordon to take a selfie outside the office to mark the occasion.

When we were called in we spoke over each other while giving the registrar our details and giggled as we answered emphatically that no, we were not related, and no, we had never been married before. The kind woman on the other side of the desk began to enter our names into the computer, taking the information from our birth certificates. As she typed Deirdre and Winston Merrimans' names, I felt a pang of discomfort. It didn't seem right. My parents were Ruaidhrí and Ger McSharry, so I asked if their names could be typed in instead.

I had been in situations like this many times. Why was the name on my birth certificate Merriman when my name was McSharry? Why was the name on my passport Merriman-McSharry? Which mother did they want when they asked for my mother's maiden name? Official forms and I had never been great friends.

Sure enough, when the kind lady came back, it was to tell me that we weren't going to be able to get our licence after all. Because I had been adopted, my birth certificate was null and void. I would have to come back with what she referred to as my 'American birth cert'. It wasn't a big deal, she assured me. I couldn't make eye contact with either her or Gordon, choosing instead to gaze out the window in an attempt to stop the prickling in my eyes.

When we got outside the office, the tears began to fall and I started to feel like an idiot. I knew the situation could be sorted with relative ease, but I was just so sick of everything being complicated. Nothing in my bloody life had ever been straightforward, so why had I ever thought I'd manage this with ease? I had been in this position so many times, and I felt a real sense of frustration. Just once, I wanted things to be normal. I felt embarrassed and, in all honesty, jealous of Gordon and his beautiful family and the simplicity with which he had been able to live his life.

I never managed to muster up any interest in planning my wedding. As the Big Day drew closer I found myself almost rebelling against the excitement. I refused to become thrilled when I collected my wedding dress, hanging it up in my room and not looking at it again until the eve of the ceremony, when I hung it up in my hotel room. I cut short a last-minute shopping trip for 'bits and bobs' because I just couldn't be arsed. When my sisters got into an argument about who was going to walk down the aisle first, I told them I really didn't care. 'Do whatever, it's not important.' And it wasn't important.

I remained fairly casual about the whole event until a minute before the ceremony started. The enormity of it finally hit me as I began to walk, arm in arm with my dad, towards all the people I love in my life. Our ceremony was outside, and there was quite a long walk from the building to the aisle, during which all eyes were on me. When I saw everyone, I squeezed my dad's arm. 'Oh my God, it's my wedding. *It's my*

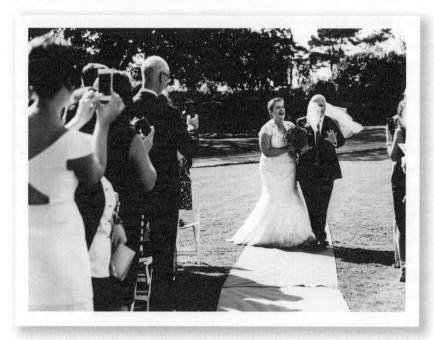

wedding! My *wedding!*' Whatever disconnection I had felt to the event disappeared when he told me to take a deep breath and slow down. I did my best, but it was only when my veil flew off my head and into his face that the tension broke. I started laughing and I didn't stop for the rest of the day. I was deliriously happy. I married the best man I know, and we had a beautiful ceremony, during which we giggled and held hands and were overwhelmed with joy.

....

When I saw everyone, I squeezed my dad's arm. 'Oh my God, it's my wedding. It's my wedding! My wedding!'

....

As it turns out, the wedding was perfect. It was everything I wanted, even if I hadn't really known what that was. I may have not been your typical bride in the run-up to the event, but now, afterwards, I am full of clichés. It was the best day of my life. I didn't want it to end. I wish we could do it again. Now I'd talk about it to anyone who would listen.

The dress

For many women, their wedding dress is something they've spent years dreaming about. They drape their granny's net curtains around themselves in childhood, surreptitiously buy bridal magazines and fold down the corner of the pages with the dresses they like as teens and, no matter what their relationship status is as adults, they trawl wedding websites looking at photos. I was not one of those people. However, having watched countless rom-coms and television programmes, I knew what to expect from shopping for my wedding dress.

First, the shops would be elegantly lit to make you look your most beautiful. The shop assistants would fall over themselves to tell you how gorgeous you looked. Every dress would be magnificent and you really wouldn't know how to choose just one. Oh, and of course your mother and bridesmaids would be there weeping at the sheer sight of you.

If you have bought a wedding dress you are probably already laughing and shaking your head because, as it turns out, this fantasy of wedding-dress shopping is bullshit. I'm sorry to shatter the illusion for you women who have not yet purchased a wedding dress, but I think it's important that you know. I think it's important that everyone knows, because for many women the experience is horrific, and it shouldn't be.

In a sea of 'shedding for the wedding' articles it may be difficult to believe, but not everyone starves themselves for their Big Day. However, when you visit a wedding-dress shop, they will only have one size in each dress. That means you will almost always be trying on potentially the most important (and most expensive) item of clothing you will ever buy in the wrong size. That is, of course, if you get to try it on at all – because if the sample is a ten and you are an eighteen, then that dress will have to be ruled out entirely. It won't matter if it's your dream dress – your options will be limited to dresses that come in a size that actually fits on your body. If you're a size eighteen to twenty – like I was when I went wedding-dress shopping – you will be able to choose from dresses that come in a sample-size sixteen and above. The rest of them won't get over your hips.

The sample will have been tried on by countless women before you and, in many cases, it'll look that way. It may well be a grimy grey instead of the original colour. There may be fake-tan marks, make-up stains and snags. Not to mention the sweat marks – because the whole thing is a sweaty experience. For the most part, wedding-dress shops are relatively small and during busy periods will have a few different people trying on dresses at the same time, leading to increased temperatures.

So picture the scenario: you are in this cramped hothouse struggling to get into a grubby dress that's one to four sizes too small for you. (And when I say 'struggling to get into', I mean that a determined member of staff is wrestling you into the garment using various straps and panels of fabric to protect your modesty.) It's no surprise, really, that when you tumble out of the changing room, dripping with sweat and struggling to breathe, you don't necessarily get the tearful reaction you had hoped for from your loved ones.

Picture the scenario: you are in this cramped hot-house struggling to get into a grubby dress that's one to four sizes too small for you.

You find yourself in front of a mirror, squinting in an attempt to imagine what the dress might look like if it was clean and if it fit you, and trying to ignore the voice in the back of your head wailing, 'Where did it all go wrong?' It's not exactly the dream.

And that's without taking into consideration the things people say to you. I was lucky and the staff in the shops I went to were lovely, and the crew filming for the documentary managed to keep any unkind remarks to themselves. However, others have had a different experience. Countless women I know have been sniffed at in shops and told that they'll have to lose a lot of weight even to consider trying on certain dresses. Can you imagine that? Imagine standing, vulnerable, in a dress that doesn't fit you, exposed and stressed, only to be told by a snooty woman that you're 'going to need to tone up those arms'? I have heard so many horror stories – some of them about very well-known and well-respected shops – that I have to wonder what the hell we're doing, putting up with such a load of crap during one of the most expensive transactions of our lives.

The first time I went shopping for my dress, everything was wrong. I've never really enjoyed shopping – hardly surprising, since I've spent most of my life feeling rejected by the shops – so I wasn't that into the idea of going wedding-dress shopping. I was worried I'd go to a shop and they wouldn't have my size. I was worried the shop assistant would look me up and down and shake her head the way the woman in the school-uniform shop did when I was fifteen. I don't ever put myself in those situations any more, and I didn't relish the idea of doing it in the context of my wedding. The anxiety I felt about this situation is exactly the reason I bang on so much about what it's like to be a plus-size woman. I don't think it's fair that I couldn't think about shopping for a wedding dress without being paralysed by fear.

Since time was ticking and I needed to get moving, my maid of honour and best friend extraordinaire told me she'd make some phone calls and organize an appointment somewhere one Saturday that would definitely have my size. Sarah organized the appointment in a shop that sold lots and lots of styles and sizes.

I had had chemo five days earlier. By rights, I should have been reasonably well by then, but a last-minute interview I'd agreed to give on *The Late Late Show* the night before had scuppered that. (The news of my cancer had recently come out and doing the interview seemed like a good way of dealing with the media interest in one go.) I was exhausted and when we arrived at the shop, camera crew in tow, I couldn't help but feel I'd made a huge mistake.

I did my best to plaster a smile on my face as I looked around the showroom, feeling extremely conspicuous after the previous night's television appearance. I didn't want to seem ungrateful for the effort Sarah had put into organizing the appointment, or to disappoint my sisters and mom, who were with me. The whole thing felt weird. I didn't feel like a bride. I didn't really know what I wanted. And since shopping with other people was not something I usually did, I felt like I was playing a role.

The women in the shop couldn't have been nicer, but when I started trying dresses on I felt horrendous. The chemo hot sweats were upon me as I struggled into them. They didn't fit me, and flashbacks of other dressing-room moments filled with self-loathing flooded my brain. How many times had I tried things on in shops only to find that I was too fat (too lazy, too repulsive)? How many times and, still, here I was? I was angry because I was gaining weight during chemo. I was angry because I *still* wasn't the skinny person I had dreamed of being for years.

Not wanting to upset anyone, I left the dressing room feeling sweaty, ashamed and embarrassed. I did not get the 'ooh's' and 'aah's' I had watched others get on TV. When I looked in the mirror, I saw a sweaty bald woman in an ill-fitting dress. Probably because I *was* a sweaty, bald woman in an ill-fitting dress. We agreed this wasn't the one. I tried another. Again: I looked sweaty and bald, and the dress was ill-fitting.

I was embarrassed. I was embarrassed that I was sweaty, embarrassed that I didn't look right, embarrassed that I wasn't giving these lovely women the reaction they wanted.

I was angry that I was exhausted. Angry that I was bald. Angry that I was having to do this all during chemo. For the first and only time during my experience with cancer, I felt really pissed off that I was going through it. It all felt very unfair.

The experience was so unpleasant that upon leaving the shop I decreed that I was *never* going wedding-dress shopping again. Nobody argued with me. For the next couple of months I simply ignored the fact that I would have to get a wedding dress. In January I spent some time in hospital and one of the nurses on the ward told me about the wonderful experience she'd had choosing her dress. The people in the shop sounded kind and welcoming and when she told me its name I realized it was just down the street from my house – ninety steps maximum – so I had to give it a go.

When I got out of hospital I emailed the shop and arranged an appointment for the following week. I told no one; I figured that if I went on my own there would be less pressure. In the end, my friend Justyne happened to be around that day so she came with me. The atmosphere in the shop was

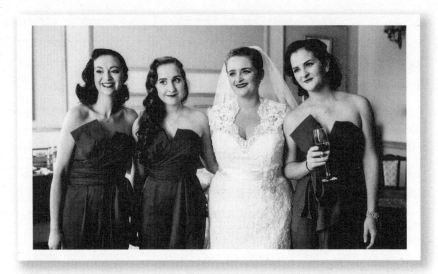

On the day, I loved my dress, and everything else about my wedding. My bridesmaids are (left to right) my best friend, Sarah, and my sisters, Aoife and Úna.

lovely. Despite having no expectations, I found several dresses that I really liked and one that I loved. A week later I returned to the shop with my mom and bridesmaids and placed my order. I can't even begin to tell you how relieved I was. I didn't have to think about it again until I had a fitting, which was months away.

When I went for my first dress fitting I was really scared. I hadn't seen the dress in seven months and I was worried that (a) I wouldn't like it and (b) it wouldn't fit. These are the three things I thought about it:

I am not thin but this looks great on me.

I look beautiful.

I can't wait to wear it.

If your wedding dress doesn't make you feel like you're beautiful and you can't wait to wear it, then you shouldn't buy it.

The jitters

Being sick of talking about the wedding itself was not the only challenge I faced in the run-up to our wedding. I got cold feet. Very cold feet.

Because I'd been sick for the whole winter, I had planned a lot for us to do in the summer. As a result, Gordon and I were extremely busy in the months before our wedding and rarely had a moment alone together. When we did find a moment, it was generally rushed and a bit cranky; often there was a terse exchange over someone not doing what they needed to around some logistical wedding issue, or not bothering to clean out the cats' litter trays. Let's say we weren't our best selves.

As the wedding came closer, the combination of the strained atmosphere and the seriousness with which I knew we were both taking our upcoming vows resulted in immense pressure. I found myself worrying constantly about whether or not we were doing the right thing. We had always got along like a house on fire, but now we weren't. What if this was it? What if we'd just hit that point relationships hit when things are no longer good? What if we got married and then realized it had all been a big mistake? Why did anyone get married anyway? How could anyone make that commitment?

What if we got married and then realized it had all been a big mistake? How could anyone promise to love someone for ever?

How could anyone promise to love someone for ever? Who knew what was right around the corner?

Outwardly, I did my best to carry on as normal but, inwardly, my anxiety was building. Every night I dreamed that I had done something to destroy our relationship, frequently to do with infidelity. I'd wake up in a sweat with new worries. *What if I cheat on him?* (I've never cheated on anyone.) *What if I break his heart?* It became clear that this was what I was really worried about. What if I hurt or disappointed this man that I loved?

What if I fuck it up? I found myself wondering, several times an hour. I struggled to act normal while people chatted to me about the wedding. *Maybe there shouldn't even be a wedding,* I'd be thinking.

A couple of weeks before the wedding, I blurted it all out while having breakfast with my mother. I explained my fears through tears, and panic, while shoving sausages into my gob. (I do my best crying while eating.) She was sympathetic but didn't seem to be taking my concerns too seriously. She pointed out that all my concerns were for Gordon's well-being and that this was a good sign rather than a bad one. Then she encouraged me to talk to him about how I was feeling.

I didn't know how to do that, and that was one of the most difficult things about the whole thing. I always told Gordon everything, and it felt absolutely horrible to be keeping something like this a secret from him. However, how did you tell someone you loved you were worried that getting married to them might be a mistake?

The next morning Ger texted me to say that she didn't have any doubts about Gordon and me. She said beautiful things about our relationship and the way we were together, and that she felt sure I was doing the right thing. Of course, I started crying as I read it, in bed. Of course, Gordon wanted to know what had me in floods.

Out it came. I explained my fears, and how I'd been feeling. How I didn't know any more if marriage was a good idea for anyone because how can you promise to be with and love someone for ever? He laughed at me a bit. In a nice way. He told me that of course no one can be certain of for ever, but that he loved me and I loved him and that we were going to be okay.

I can't even tell you how it felt as the weight lifted off my shoulders. I knew that everything was going to be all right. I

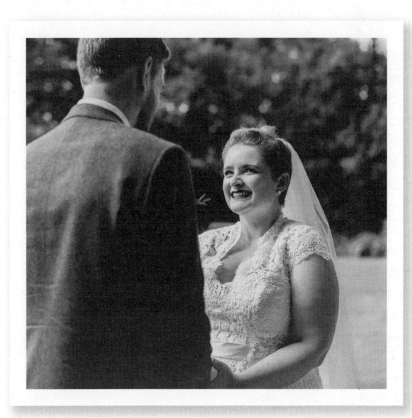

felt entirely foolish for letting this train of thought run around my brain for so long on its own. It seemed stupid not to have just spoken it out loud and nipped it in the bud at an earlier stage. Everything was easier once you'd said it out loud – I knew that! Anyway, we hugged and got on with it and, on our wedding day, I didn't have a single doubt. In fact, I was entirely confident. I still am.

Kids

I have always wanted kids. You don't really need a degree in psychology to figure out that this desire probably partly stems from my complicated family background. I've always felt a strong desire to create what I didn't have. A family with two parents who loved each other. A family where I felt safe. A family where my children felt loved, all the time. When I say it like that it sounds like I want to have kids to fix my past, which probably isn't great, but at the core of it is a desire to be a mother. A good one.

I don't just want the kids either. I want to be pregnant. I want to take a pregnancy test and marvel at how gross it is to hold a stick I've just urinated on in my hand. I want to wave said urine-soaked stick in Gordon's face and watch his face as he realizes what it means. I want to walk around with a secret that only we know about until we feel it's safe to tell people. I want to nurture my baby as it grows inside of me and panic over whether or not I've ruined it with that glass of wine I had when I didn't realize I was pregnant. I want to gain weight in places I didn't think I could and have trouble sleeping because I'm so huge. I want to feel my baby kick. I want to give birth and experience the all-consuming pain that millions of women have felt before me. I want to be pregnant. I want the good, I want the bad. I want the lot.

I want to be pregnant. I want the good, I want the bad. I want the lot.

I've never taken the idea of getting pregnant for granted. Even when I was fearfully taking a pregnancy test in the toilets of the UCD arts block there was a part of me that thought, 'Well, at least I'd know that I can get pregnant.' As a result, when it came time for me to have chemo and therefore deal with the fertility risks that come with it, I found myself saying, 'Well, who knows? Maybe I already had fertility problems? There's no point in worrying about it.' The doctors and nurses reassured me that the type of chemo I would be receiving was not the worst for female fertility and that they'd had plenty of patients who'd had healthy babies afterwards. They gave me an injection called Decapeptyl anyway, which would encourage my ovaries to take cover during the onslaught of poisonous drugs my body was about to face. 'The idea is that they'll uncover again once the chemo has finished,' an endocrinologist told me in his office. 'And, you know, there's some evidence that it works.' I giggled nervously and repeated this story to friends afterwards. 'There's *some* evidence that it works,' I'd laugh. 'How very comforting!'

I would never have considered myself to be a particularly positive person, but when it came to serious medical situations I always just assumed that everything would be grand. I had done so in the run-up to my jaunt with cancer and, despite being wrong on that occasion, I felt the same way approaching post-chemo fertility testing. I thought I'd be fine. I really did.

The first bit of doubt crept in when I went to meet my friend Sarah for an on-camera chat as part of filming for my RTÉ documentary. I had met Sarah in the hospital during treatment and instantly felt drawn to her. Some people are just magnetic, and from the minute I saw her I wanted to know more. She had the cancer look that loads of us had in the unit – no eyebrows, no hair, zero eyelashes – but she was shining. I forced my way into the conversation she was having with our shared specialist nurse, and that night she added me on Facebook. Although she was seventeen and I was thirty-one we became friends. Cancer is the truest equalizer I've ever encountered, and the age gap has never felt relevant.

I knew she'd be perfect for the documentary because she is so articulate and funny, and unbelievably mature. It was her maturity that disarmed me as we sat in her mam's kitchen and she told me that she had learned she was essentially infertile as a result of chemotherapy. I couldn't believe that vibrant, young Sarah had been dealt this blow. It just seemed so very unfair. And then the selfish thoughts crept in. If it had happened to her, it could happen to me.

It could happen to me.

The next time I saw my consultant I asked for a referral to a fertility specialist. Gordon and I had been discussing when we might like to have a baby. I was keen to get going, but Gordon wanted a little more playtime before we settled down properly. It seemed like a smart thing to do to find out where we were in terms of our fertility and to have all the information. If we needed to, we could start trying straight away; if not, we could take our time.

We visited the fertility unit in the Rotunda Hospital at the end of April, almost three months after my last chemo treatment. The doctor was enthusiastic and direct in a way we found amusing, and arranged for us to give the required samples. For me, it meant getting blood taken on the day. For Gordon, things were a bit more awkward and, like a scene from a film, he found himself cycling a sample in to the hospital on his bike, keeping 'his sperms', as we called them, warm in his jacket pocket. We laughed about it and the likely futility of all this rigmarole. We'd be fine!

We were due to get the results about six weeks later. I didn't think about it much in the interim, aside from mentioning it in passing to friends over coffee, joking that the appointment was the day before our girls' trip to Ibiza. 'If it's bad news' – hilarious grimace – 'well, I'll need a drink for sure!'

On the day itself my close friends asked me how I felt. I told them I felt fine. I did. I was sure it would all be okay. 'I've been grand so far, so there's no reason to believe this will be any different' was the line I was spinning, and I felt it, too, right up until I found myself in the waiting room for my appointment. The walls of the room are covered in facts about the unit itself and IVF in general. I found myself wondering if I would need to have IVF, and then pondering adoption. Would I be able to adopt? What if I didn't love the child? What if it grew up to be really bold? Or ... ugly? Could I love it? I scolded myself internally for such terrible thoughts and gave myself a good talking-to. *You're going to be fine. Stop being such a drama queen.* After a few minutes Gordon and I were brought up from the main waiting room to a small internal one, where I explained the rules of the game show on the television to him. 'It's like *Eggheads*, but true or false. The expert people don't seem as dickheady as the ones on *Eggheads*, though.' We hadn't ever really discussed what might happen if this appointment didn't go well, and we weren't about to do it then. We were going to be fine. I was sure of it. Until I saw the doctor.

*

I would never have predicted that I would come to a point in my life where I could recognize the look a doctor gets on their face when they're about to give you bad news, but that is exactly where I find myself now. It's a particular face, the bad-news one. It's kinder and softer than the usual doctor face. You can see the compassion and feel a heaviness in the air. I felt it when I was diagnosed. And I felt it in the Rotunda.

Part of me wanted to turn and run, but I went through the motions, and when he said, 'I'm afraid it's not good news,' I sat trying to manage myself because, even in these situations where it's perfectly appropriate to cry, you really mustn't. The doctor explained that Gordon's 'little guys' were fine but that chemotherapy had essentially decimated my egg supply. Where a woman my age should be between thirty and forty on the scale they use to measure fertility, I was at two.

'It's not all doom and gloom,' the doctor said, passing me a box of tissues when a few of my tears betrayed me by spilling down my cheeks. 'It's not impossible.' He told me stories of various patients who had beaten the odds and got pregnant naturally. He told us that, as soon as my haematologist approved, we should start trying and, if it didn't happen in the next eighteen months, then we could reassess. Oh, but I'd need to lose a good bit of weight if I wanted IVF. (*Thanks a million, doctor. Thank you so much. That is exactly what I need to hear right now.*)

Gordon asked a few questions, but I absolutely had to get out of there. I said the right things – 'Well, there's nothing we can do, so we'll just have to give it a go and hope for the best' – and politely rejected the offer of some emotional support from the nice ladies who serve that purpose in the hospital.

As soon as I could, I made a mad dash for the door, wanting to leave that place and the very nice people who worked there very firmly behind.

As the door closed after me, the sobbing began, and I stood there in the car park of the Rotunda, on a beautiful sunny day, hating everything around me. I hated this bloody hospital. Hated every woman in it for being pregnant and having a baby. Hated bloody chemotherapy, and hated my bloody body for failing me.

> *I hated this bloody hospital. Hated every woman in it for being pregnant and having a baby. Hated bloody chemotherapy, and hated my bloody body for failing me.*

I could barely look at Gordon. I could never just be simple, could I? Things always had to be complicated. He, who had never given me a moment of trouble, was facing down the barrel of yet another gun because – yet again – there was a problem with me. He had cycled to the appointment, so we said temporary goodbyes and went our separate ways; he out the side gate with his bike and me through the baby-filled hospital to the bus stop across the road.

I was seething and failing entirely to control my tears as I looked at the pregnant women smoking outside the hospital and thinking all the horribly judgemental things I try my best not to think. On my bus there were not one but two teenage girls with buggies, and again I thought all the terrible things I really should not have thought. I turned my face to the window as I wept silently, trying to avoid the gaze of three addicts sitting near me. I didn't want to enter into any conversation, and tears are a demon for that. All I wanted was to go home, get into my bed and cry bitterly until I couldn't cry any more. I did not feel positive. I did not feel rational. I was raging.

'Please don't tell anyone yet,' I said to Gordon. I couldn't face the idea of his parents, two good people who had raised a man who was generous and kind, knowing that I was making things difficult once more. I felt like a complete failure.

You're probably thinking all the kind things people think when someone is being a bit hard on themselves. If you were here with me you'd fall over yourself to comfort me, and tell me about all the people you know who struggled with fertility but went on to beat the odds. If I were you, I'd do the same. At the time, however, there was no room for reason and there was literally nothing anyone could say to comfort me.

I found myself questioning the value of chemotherapy. Wondering if I'd even needed it. Thinking the whole thing had probably been blown out of proportion. I should never have had it in the first place. Even if it was necessary, was there even any point if it meant I couldn't have a baby? I was not in a good place. Even in the context of all that darkness, though, that really annoying sensible voice was coming through.

People go through this all the time, Louise.

You're at two, not zero. You should be grateful for that.

You're lucky to have made it this far without complications.

Sometimes, I hate that stupid voice. I really wanted to wallow, but I couldn't while that reasonable voice was annoying me in my head, so I got out of bed and started packing for Ibiza.

By the time I got home from my few days away I felt strong enough to tell my parents about the results. The conversations felt oddly similar to those I'd had nine months earlier when I told them I had cancer. Once again, I felt I needed to manage their reactions. I needed to keep the conversations short and to assure them that everything would be okay.

I have no choice but to believe that it will be okay. That I will one day pee on a stick and be thrilled at the result.

Like with the cancer, the more I said that things would be okay, the more I believed it, and now I have comforted myself into a corner where I have no choice but to believe that it will be okay. That the few eggs I have left are going to work. That I will one day pee on a stick and be thrilled at the result. Anything else is unthinkable.

I always thought I'd have a baby at thirty-four. The goo came upon me in my late twenties, but thirty-four seemed like the right age. Hopefully, I'd be in a good place in my career by then. Hopefully, I'd have got wild nights and lost weekends out of my system. Hopefully, Gordon would be ready.

With things as they are now, it seems ludicrous to have picked an age. I always knew on some level that it was silly. 'I know you can't plan these things,' I'd say. But I was still planning.

Now I spend all my time thinking about how lucky I'll be if I manage it by then. Gone are the conversations about whether we should have three children or four. Instead, I think about what it would be like to have one little baby in my arms. My eyes fill with tears when I think about just how much we would love him or her. How Gordon would look while he held our baby, not just what he would look like but the look in his eyes. The love. I want it so badly that a lot of the time I have to stop myself from going there and instead force myself to imagine what it will be like if it doesn't happen. That would be okay, too. *That would be okay, too.*

Now that we're actively trying, I find myself in the strange position of desperately wanting to get pregnant and also hoping that it doesn't happen straight away. I want to go to Glastonbury again. I want another summer of fun. But then I know that if I am at Glastonbury in the summer of 2016 then it probably means that it's not going to happen. It means IVF. Egg donation. Adoption. Thousands of euro and years of hoping, working and waiting. Years of disappointment. I know women go through it all the time, and I find myself feeling their pain at a very deep level. It seems so cruel that we spend so much of our lives doing everything we can to avoid pregnancy only to find out at a later stage that it's not an option anyway. Surely there's a better way. Surely we can save ourselves some of the pain.

Gordon says he's ready now. On one hand, it's a relief. When the fertility specialist told us we should start trying, I felt guilty. I was rushing him into it. He didn't have a choice. At least I know he wants it. Now, though, I have a different reason to feel guilty. He's ready now. And I probably can't make it happen for him.

Since speaking publicly about my issues, lovely people are keen to tell me about their sister or neighbour or friend who was told she'd never have children but now has 'three healthy kids'. I know they mean well. I know the intentions are good. But my head says, 'They're the exception.' I smile at the people and say, 'Yes, sure. Hopefully, it'll be grand,' and then

I change the subject. In the context of these exceptions, I see only another opportunity for me to fail.

My friends who have babies feel guilty now for saying a bad word about motherhood. 'Sorry, I shouldn't be saying this to you,' they say as they hold their little ones. I tell them not to worry, and I mean it. I don't feel envious of them, which is strange, because I've been envious of people my whole life. I hope it can stay that way. I can imagine that if you've been trying to get pregnant for a long time and it's not happening, bitterness might creep in. Now, though, I just feel really happy for anyone who's managed to do it. It's almost like if I can just be good enough, kind enough, loving enough, then maybe I will be rewarded for it. Maybe I can join their club.

Currently, I'm in a club whose members number in the thousands. I am one of many women who find themselves trying for a baby while knowing that they probably won't be successful. The reality of being in the club is challenging.

> **I'm in a club whose members number in the thousands. I am one of many women who find themselves trying for a baby while knowing that they probably won't be successful. The reality of being in the club is challenging.**

You download your fertility app of choice and mark down the days of your cycle. It sends you push notifications, asking you whether or not you have anything to report. You don't.

You make sure you have sex on the days marked green, because these are the days on which a normal woman has a twenty per cent chance of getting pregnant rather than a two per cent chance of getting pregnant. You know, though, that you are not normal and therefore those percentages do not apply to you. But you make sure you remind your partner that it's a key day in your cycle and that you have to have sex on that day. You get a push notification reminding you of this fact.

You manage to have sex once that day. It's weird, because you both know what it's really about and the spontaneity is gone. You go to sleep feeling like you really should have managed it twice at the very least. You're really not doing enough if you want to beat the odds.

You feel strangely tired so you google 'tiredness and pregnancy'. Apparently, you are very tired during early pregnancy, so maybe you're pregnant. Your inner voice tells you you're not, but a small flame of hope is ignited. You get a touch of thrush. You google 'thrush and early pregnancy'. Apparently, some women experience it in early pregnancy. The flame is fed. You start to calculate the months. If you are pregnant now, then when will you have the baby? What will the baby look like? You know you should get a grip because you're very probably not pregnant, but you can't help but imagine what it would be like to hold your little baby in your arms.

Weeks pass, and your app tells you that you should be getting your period. Your period has never been particularly regular but still the flame of hope grows. You start to wonder if you should take a test, but then you tell yourself that would be stupid and you can't take a test every time you convince yourself you might be pregnant because the doctor has told you it's probably not going to happen, so who are you kidding?

You go to sleep and dream you are taking a pregnancy test and it's positive, and you are delighted. All the jokes you've been making about wanting to get pregnant but also wanting to go to Glastonbury are ridiculous, because you really want to get pregnant. In the dream you take another test, and another. They are positive. Dream You tells your dream husband that you've taken seventeen pregnancy tests and they're all positive, but Dream You can't quite believe that it's true. Dream You takes one final test while your dream husband waits outside the toilet, but when you look at the test it's all red, and negative, because you've got your period. Dream You is heartbroken. You wake up and Real You is heartbroken.

You are facing into months and possibly years of this. You don't know if you can take it. You decide to take a test. You buy the test. It's negative. The next day, you get your period. You enter it into the app and start again.

7
Family

Dee and me

The day I finished my Leaving Cert in June 2000 my dad gave me a lift to a friend's house to get ready for our big night out. I was excited, delighted to be off the leash and looking forward to celebrating, but after a couple of minutes he turned to me and said some of the most terrifying words a person can hear: 'I need to tell you something.'

Dee had been in touch. We hadn't seen or heard from her since before we left the States three years earlier. In fact, I had only seen her once since the incident on the street when she had humiliated me in front of my friends. We met her by chance about nine months afterwards. Ger, Andrew, Úna and I were going for a walk along the Fox River, and there she was. She was sober, but miserable. She seemed embarrassed and ashamed. Before I would have done anything I could to comfort her. This time, I resisted. I think I had really just had enough. Enough hurt. Enough disappointment. I was done with the apologies I had accepted so readily in the past. I was done excusing her.

For this reason, our last encounter was burned into my brain. For the first time ever, I hadn't let her off the hook. I can still feel the ache in my chest when I picture her face looking at me pleadingly as I told her that what she'd done that day was really not okay.

In the intervening years I had thought about her often. I had wondered if I would ever see her again and concluded that I probably wouldn't. I thought the most likely turn of events would be that I would hear she had died in tragic circumstances. I had hardened myself in anticipation of that news. I was not ready to hear that not only had she been in touch but she was sober. And paralysed.

My dad told me they had decided to wait until I finished my exams to tell me she'd been in contact, and he encouraged me to take what she had to say with a pinch of salt. After years and years of lying and manipulation, it was hard for him to trust her. I often think that regaining people's trust must be one of the hardest parts of recovery for an addict. When you've spent decades hurting and disappointing people, it takes time to get them back onside.

> *Regaining people's trust must be one of the hardest parts of recovery for an addict. When you've spent decades hurting and disappointing people, it takes time to get them back onside.*

I was reeling when I got out of my dad's car. I explained the situation to my friend, but she didn't get it. 'I don't know why you care about her any more, after all she did to you,' she said.

What she didn't understand was that, for years, we'd been a team, me and Dee. As sick and unhealthy as it is, it felt like we'd been partners – us against the world. Sometimes that meant I felt unbelievably safe as she cuddled me on the couch in front of the fire, and sometimes it meant lying to someone about the bottle of vodka hidden in the cistern. But it was always us two. Losing that will always be with me.

On that night, I was confused. The little girl in me wondered if this was it: had I got my wish and Dee was sober and we could be together? The grown-up in me was scared.

Could I believe it? Was she really off the booze? What would this mean for my life?

As it turned out, Ruaidhrí's and my doubts were unfounded. Dee was telling the truth. She *was* sober. She had been sober for about eight months. During this time she had been diagnosed with bipolar disorder, which explained those moments of excitement so intense that she got us up in the middle of the night to share them with her. And then there was her paralysis. After we lost contact with her, things in her life had taken a dark turn. Well, darker. She became homeless, living under a bridge through freezing Chicago winters. She hung out with a group of guys. A group of guys who ended up being responsible for a beating so bad she couldn't walk any more.

Still that wasn't her turning point. Dee kept drinking. I can understand that: if alcohol is the only thing you believe can get you through the day and you experience an extreme trauma, why the hell would you stop? She did stop, though, and, as she tells it, she stopped in the most unlikely of circumstances. She was at a barbecue, with free beer, when she turned to a friend and said, 'Take me to the emergency room.' Once she was there she told them she was an alcoholic and was having suicidal thoughts, and then she fought for treatment. The first place she went was too easy, she says. She knew she was too smart for it. She needed somewhere tough. She heard about a place which sounded right for her, but there were no spaces available. She rang them every day until they let her in. She wouldn't take no for an answer.

I feel incredibly proud when I think of her doing that. Not only was she seeking help but she was seeking help that would work. She knew that, if she went into a touchy-feely, nicey-nicey place, she'd start drinking again. She needed somewhere that would be hard on her, and when she found it she made it happen. She worked it, and it worked.

Dee came to Ireland the following year. I was so excited about seeing her. Now that I was an adult I wanted to see if I'd grown into a body that was similar to hers. I wanted to ask her if she got period pains and to see if her hands looked like mine. At times as a teenage girl, I'd found it hard not to have my biological mother. That's no shade on Ger, who did her very best, but sometimes, when your hormones are raging and everything in life seems unfair, you think you need your bio-mom.

Our reunion was joyful and babbling. I was so happy to see her, and to see her sober, that my eyes glossed over the wheelchair. I just wouldn't think about it. I wouldn't think about what had happened to her. I wouldn't allow myself to be upset about it. We hung out for a while and met up a couple more times during her trip. But over the weeks my feelings started to change. My initial delight at seeing her gave way to anger, and by the end of her stay I wanted to scream when people complimented her for turning things around.

'Isn't your mother great, Louise?' relatives said. In my head I was going, '*She's not my mother!*' I found all this praise she was getting difficult to listen to and felt protective of Ger. Ger had made the sacrifices. Ger had done the hard work. Ger was the one I had yelled, '*I hate you!*' at countless times during my teenage years, and who had done everything she

> **I felt protective of Ger. Ger had made the sacrifices. Ger was my mother. Ger is my mother.**

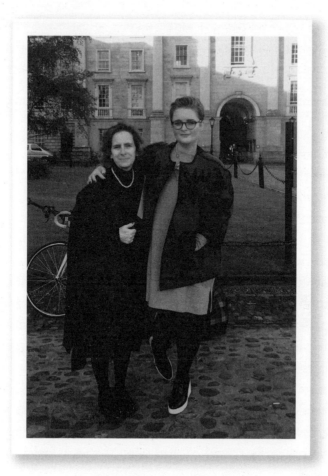

*At Trinity with my mom, Ger, at her
third graduation. November 2015.*

could to keep me safe, though we were related only by marriage. Ger was my mother. Ger *is* my mother.

When Dee went back to Chicago I stopped communicating
with her and began a pattern which continues to this day. It's
not her fault. She has done her best. When she came back to
Ireland two years after that initial visit, she let me roar and

shout at her. She has answered all the questions I can ask to the best of her ability. (For instance, she's the one who told me that she knew my father died worrying about her drinking: a hard thing for her to admit and a horrible thing for me to think about – how those worries must have added to his distress as he was dying.) She has done her best to stay in touch, sending me emails, even when I don't respond for months.

I can't really explain why I have such a hard time communicating with her. I keep saying I'm not angry with her but, on some level, I must be. I think I'm angry at her for not being the mom I knew when I was little, the good mom, though she can't possibly be. I think I blame who she is now for taking away the person who was so familiar to me.

I've worked on it, and thought about it and spoken to therapists about it. Every time I think I'm okay I find myself again resisting a relationship with her. I stop communicating. Then I feel guilty. Then I resent feeling guilty. Then I feel angry at her for making me feel guilty and resentful.

In recent years she has visited Dublin twice a year for several weeks, at Christmas and in the summertime. She always sends me emails ahead of her visits, expressing a desire to meet up, 'hopefully more than once this time'. I don't always reply. In fact, I rarely answer her emails and when I do my responses are cursory. Again, I'm not proud of that, but it is the reality.

During her visits she contacts me several times in an attempt to arrange a rendezvous and, generally, just before she goes home, I meet her for dinner, always with Gordon. Gordon is an amazing person to have in any situation you feel even slightly awkward about. He has a gift for putting people at ease and can chat effortlessly to anyone in any scenario. (I sometimes think that being with him has been bad for my social skills, because I can just sit back and relax while he runs the show.) I always feel anxious ahead of these meetings with Dee, and afterwards Gordon always says, 'Well, that was okay, wasn't it?' And it is always okay. And it is always a relief that it's done for another six months or so.

Usually, I am able to articulate my feelings about this sort of thing easily, but on this matter I always struggle. Perhaps even I am not entirely clear why I feel the way I do. On paper, I am filled with admiration for her. What she has done to turn her life around is incredible. Since getting sober, she has returned to college and got a Ph.D. She has volunteered with a rape crisis network. She is somehow involved with the bloody UN! So I guess the answer to the question 'Isn't your mother great, Louise?' is yes. For some reason, I just struggle with it.

The truth is that I don't really know where she belongs in my life now. She is not my mother. She is not my friend. I don't know what this relationship is supposed to look like. If you imagine having someone in your life who you don't feel you know very well but who has a very intense interest in you and every element of your life, you might be able to imagine where I'm coming from. She yearns for more from me, and I fail her every time.

So I'm glad she lives in Chicago. I'm glad of the distance. I don't feel good saying that, but that's how it is. I struggle to find a role for her in my life now. She has a lifetime of love for me but it only makes me uncomfortable. The fact is that I never stopped being her daughter but she stopped being my mother twenty-five years ago.

> *I never stopped being her daughter but she stopped being my mother twenty-five years ago.*

While I'm not angry with her in the way that some people expect me to be, I don't feel any real compulsion to be close to her either.

Sometimes I think my brother took the right route. When Dee got back in touch with us, he had no interest in being in touch with her. Again, it wasn't because he was angry, it was because he felt he had parents and he didn't really need another parental relationship. For twelve years, that was that. A couple of years ago we were at a reunion of sorts at my parents' and he had a short conversation with Dee, in which she asked if she could have his email address. He said yes, and went on, 'But I probably won't respond.' He was honest. He is not trapped in a back and forth in which he constantly feels like he's letting someone down.

Almost immediately after Gordon and I got engaged people started asking me whether or not I would invite Dee to the wedding. I thought about it, but it seemed obvious to me we would. I knew it would mean a lot to her to be there, and I think it did. I was aware, however, that it would also be difficult for her to be there as a guest rather than as mother of the bride. I thought about it a lot in the run-up to the event, and I really did mean to meet her to talk about it, but it just didn't happen. Then I really meant to meet her to talk to her about it after the wedding, but I didn't do that either. So now I'm rolling down the path of guilt once more.

There is a voice in my head that tells me not to feel guilty. It tells me I'm entitled to my feelings and that I didn't ask to be put in this position and, therefore, if I never want to speak to Dee again, then that would be okay. But it's not, and that's not really what I want either. I don't know what I want. I don't know what to do. I don't know how to be in a relationship with someone who used to be my mother. I do know that I care about her. I do know that I love her. And I do know that I'm trying to figure it out, even if, so far, I've failed.

Dad

One of the most special relationships I have in my life is with my dad. One part child, one part ferocious businessman, Ruaidhrí has played a huge role in making me who I am today.

We are both obsessively punctual, though I'm a little less so than him. For years we were very early to everything, until he was given out to by my granny, his mother, who told him it was rude. From then on he arrived on the dot of the appointed time instead.

We both struggle to relax sometimes, which isn't great. I have a tendency to worry about the well-being of everyone around me, so if I think someone is uncomfortable I become uncomfortable. As a result, we are sometimes a circle of discomfort.

We share a similar point of view and tend to be on the same side of family discussions on current affairs and the like. When we sit around the dinner table, I often find that we're exchanging glances, wordlessly expressing scepticism about someone's opinion, or agreeing with each other on whatever's being debated. My sister Úna has banned the discussion of religion, but Dad and I have the same feelings about that too.

Ruaidhrí has an incredible sense of fun and spends a lot of time trying to make those around him laugh, often to Ger's detriment. My friends love him, and he enjoys them being around.

He encourages us to enjoy our lives and find our passions,

sometimes with a wistful look in his eyes. As a young person, he was very academically focused, something he regrets somewhat. Now, in his fifties, I think he's trying to make up for lost time. He's taken up painting, which he loves, and he spends many Saturdays on St Stephen's Green, selling his work. He travels to France and Italy every summer to paint with his 'art friends'.

A few Christmases ago, just when we thought the presents had all been opened, Ruaidhrí announced that there was one more. He left the sitting room and next we heard the sound of him dragging something down the hall, giggling all the way. 'What could it be?' he said as he brought a large box into the front room. I assumed it was a present for the house, something for the family to enjoy. I was wrong. It was an electric guitar. Which he had bought himself. For himself. And wrapped.

I've spent much of my life trying to impress him. When we had burritos for dinner in America, my mom used to make two versions of the filling – one mild and one spicy. The spicy one was for me and Ruaidhrí. I don't like spicy food but, if Ruaidhrí was having it, so would I. For years I played football, though I hated it, because he loves it. I even refereed for a while, because he was in charge of the local league's network of referees.

As I said, when I dropped out of UCD, the worst part of it was that I had disappointed him. He had gone to check my results while I was on holiday, only to find that I hadn't taken my exams. He phoned to speak to me about it and I could hear the hurt in his

When I dropped out of UCD, the worst part of it was that I had disappointed him. I could hear the hurt in his voice.

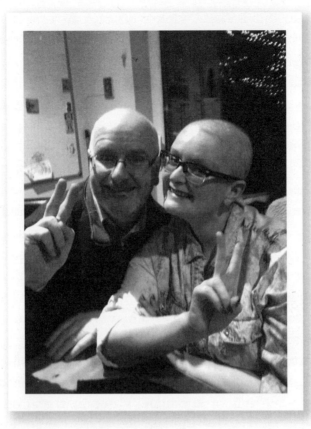

The most my Dad and I have
ever looked like each other!
Autumn 2014.

voice. I carried his sense of disappointment in me, and it was only when I started working full-time in Newstalk that I saw it go away. When he mentioned that he'd told someone I was working there, I knew the tables had turned. I was out of the doghouse.

The first time I remember truly impressing him was at a U2 concert in Croke Park. Ruaidhrí is a huge U2 fan, one of those who will tell you that he saw them right at the start, in the Dandelion Market. When he went to the States on a scholarship to do a master's, he brought his U2 records with him. They connected him to home and made him feel proud. He went on a pilgrimage to Red Rocks in Colorado, where U2 had famously filmed their *Under a Blood Red Sky* concert. He just wanted to see it.

When U2 announced they were playing gigs in Croke Park in 2005, our family was determined to go. You were only allowed to buy tickets in pairs, but we managed to get six. Two in one stand, two in another and two on the pitch. It was decided that Ruaidhrí and I would take the pitch tickets. On the day of the gig, he started texting me at 5 a.m. It began with photos from the band's gigs on the Vertigo Tour. I got about one every ten minutes until six o'clock. Then the begging started: 'When can we go?' By seven, I was up, and by eight we were in the queue outside Croke Park.

My dad likes to differentiate himself from the other 'crazy U2 fans'. He's not one of them. However, we were among them that morning. The people who queue for U2 gigs at that time of the morning are people who dedicate their lives to the band. They travel with them on tour, selling their belongings to keep them going. They wear souvenirs from other gigs as badges of honour. They have their own numerical system to ensure that people in the queue stay in the order they arrive in. It is all very serious.

It turned out to be a blisteringly hot day, and we both got sunburnt as we sat on the pavement, waiting to go in to the stadium, but when we got in we were in the pit, and it was all worth it, for Ruaidhrí to have the peace of mind of having a good spot. For me, it was worth it when I saw him react when the band came on stage. I don't have a time machine, but I certainly felt like I'd gone back in time as my dad transformed in front of my eyes. Gone was the middle-aged businessman and in his place was a seventeen-year-old boy seeing his favourite band. He knew every word to every song and sang along with gusto. He jumped up and down and reached his hands and fingers towards the stage. He was enraptured and, while I enjoyed the gig, it was his reaction that was the real show for me.

A few years later, U2 announced more dates at Croke Park, and we agreed we would stick with our routine. Ruaidhrí and I would be on the pitch and the rest of the family would be in the stand. I was living in Galway at the time and got the bus up the night before the gig. I met up with a guy I was casually seeing, and things got a little out of control. I failed to recognize the one that was one too many and when I woke up the next morning it was eight o'clock and Ruaidhrí had left without me. I'll never forget the bolt of terror that went through me when Ger told me he was gone. '*Why didn't he wake me up?*' I asked. Apparently, he had tried. I had royally fucked up.

Ignoring my hangover, I was out of the house in minutes and straight on to a bus, willing it to go faster as I imagined how disappointed Ruaidhrí would be with me. My leg bounced up and down and my heart pounded. It was so slow I abandoned it in favour of running the rest of the way to Croke Park. When I got there the queue was already quite long. I couldn't even see him. But I knew I had to get to him.

I am not someone who enjoys breaking rules. In fact, if I am knowingly doing something that goes against the guidelines, I get an overwhelming sense of anxiety. So I don't skip queues, even when I can easily get away with it. But this was different. I hopped my way up along the barrier, explaining as I went, 'I'm really sorry, I know this is awful, I just really need to get to my dad, he's here on his own and I woke up late and it's *all my fault.*' Most people allowed me to pass, the odd person tutting and shaking their head.

Finally I spotted him and it seemed like I was going to make it. There were only around twelve people between me and him. But then I hit a wall. A 300-pound Dutch wall. 'WHERE IS YOUR NUMBER?' he shouted at me, pointing at the bold, black-markered number on his hand. 'I know,' I said. 'I don't have one, and I'm really sorry, but my dad is just there and he's on his own and I just really messed up and I woke up late. I'm so sorry.'

'YOU CAN'T GET PAST IF YOU DON'T HAVE A NUMBER!' the Dutchman bellowed into my face.

'I understand,' I said, 'I know there's a system, and I would never normally do this, but I woke up late, and I really messed up, and I can't leave my dad there on his own all day.'

I pointed at my dad. At this stage, I had an audience. Everyone around us in the queue was watching, including the people sitting around my dad.

'HE IS NOT ON HIS OWN!' the Dutchman shouted, as I pleaded with him. I was not about to give up, but this man was not backing down either. Suddenly, I felt a hand reach out and yank me up the queue. The next thing I knew I was beside my dad, with the people around him applauding.

It wasn't Ruaidhrí who had pulled me up, though, it was a man who had been sitting beside him in the queue with his own daughter.

'That was ridiculous,' the stranger said. 'Some people take it too far.'

I thanked him profusely, explaining again that I had messed up and slept it out and that I just *had* to get to my dad. We sat down, and my heart rate slowly but surely returned to normal. My dad was silent as I apologized profusely to him. Eventually, he said, 'I really didn't think you'd manage that,' and for the first time in my life I saw real, true admiration in his eyes.

The gig was great, and we had a lovely time. He did his usual time-travelling bit, and we sang all the songs, but for me the real achievement that day was impressing my dad. At last.

I love that we like spending time together as adults. He's very fond of my best mate, and vice versa. He gets on well with Gordon. At my wedding, he was the star of the show. He spoke to everyone, and gave it socks on the dance floor. When the lads decided, apropos of nothing, to take their shirts off at some late stage in the evening, he joined in, much to everyone's delight.

The next day, we laughed about it, and I reminded the lads I was speaking to that, whatever about them taking their shirts off, my dad had been sober! He doesn't drink, you see. Because he's an alcoholic. He stopped drinking more than ten years ago.

It is one of the best things that has happened in my life, because, when he got sober, he changed entirely. All of the lovely things I've said about our relationship are true, but they haven't always been.

When he got sober, he changed entirely. All of the lovely things I've said about our relationship are true, but they haven't always been.

At the time Andrew and I went to live with Ruaidhrí and Ger nobody, including themselves, realized that he had a drinking problem. Initially, it seemed like he was a normal drinker. He certainly didn't drink the way Dee did; he just had a few beers or a bottle of wine after work. It was only when his drinking got in the way of our normal lives that we realized it was a problem.

I'm not sure when it happened, but at some stage Ger and he obviously made an agreement that he wouldn't drink any more. But instead of stopping the drinking, this just forced it underground. There would be weeks and weeks where he didn't drink a drop. The thing about addiction is that, even if a person isn't actively using, the addiction has taken over their brain. Unless an addict has the right tools, not using is so stressful and difficult they are on the edge at all times. So during those weeks when he was off the booze we got used to never knowing which Ruaidhrí was going to walk in the door that evening. It didn't take much to set him off and he was often not very pleasant to be around.

Úna had been born two years after we went to live with Ger and Ruaidhrí. She was adorable on the outside and inside, and we were mad about her. Ruaidhrí was besotted. I'll never forget how delighted he was when she was born. At that time, it was the happiest I'd ever seen him. But the happiness didn't last. He just couldn't resist the booze and every once in a while he would binge.

Ger did her best to shield us from it but, any time she went away, Ruaidhrí would take advantage of the opportunity to drink and I would be back in the role of parent, taking care of Andrew and Úna. I'd find myself taking her around the corner to a friend's house if he'd had a few beers.

My senses were finely tuned, and I could immediately tell if he'd been drinking. Every encounter with him began with an assessment of whether or not he was on the sauce. Most of the time, he wasn't. His ability to go for ages without booze was impressive but, when he was drinking, he'd never admit it. He would stand in front of you and lie through slurred speech and bleary eyes.

Having grown up with alcoholic parents, and having dealt with Dee, it must have been painful for him to face the fact that he was an alcoholic. I think that's why for years he restricted his drinking to night-time and the weekend. He must have been determined to convince himself he wasn't like them. Unfortunately, alcoholism doesn't discriminate, and just because your drinking hasn't resulted in you hitting your wife or losing your job doesn't mean you're not an addict.

> **Alcoholism doesn't discriminate, and just because your drinking hasn't resulted in you hitting your wife or losing your job doesn't mean you're not an addict.**

Of course, like in any family, daily life had its ups and downs. It wasn't all tension and anxiety. But the worry about Ruaidhrí's drinking was always in the background. I'm not sure any of us liked Ruaidhrí very much, no matter how much we loved him. He could sometimes be tough and incredibly cutting, which I now know was a symptom of his unhappiness.

I kind of gave up on him. I started leaving the house on Christmas Day to go to my aunt and uncle's – my biological dad's brother Greg and his wife, Linda. I didn't want to spend time at home. After one particularly awful evening I moved out and didn't speak to him for three months. Then, one night, his beloved U2 came on in the club I was in and I felt a terrible pang of missing him and met up with him the next day. We were talking again.

That was the thing about our relationship: although he was so wrapped up in his own troubles and this resulted in him being unpleasant, I always loved him. I always knew that the lovely person he is now was who he really was. I knew that the anger and tension were symptoms of an underlying problem rather than his true self.

I'm so grateful that Ruaidhrí's drinking came to a head eleven years ago. He went into residential treatment for six weeks and, when he came out, he was a different man. It sounds simplistic, but it's the truth. He was more patient. He had learned how to relax a little, which is something he'd never been able to do. Little by little, I got to know him again and began to trust that he wasn't going to drink any more. Little by little, we rebuilt our relationship. Little by little, I got to the point where I believed I could rely on him. Where I couldn't do without him. Where we could hug and say we loved each other, something we would never have done before he got sober.

A few months in advance of the wedding I played Ruaidhrí the song I wanted playing as we walked down the aisle together. It's 'All the Ways You Wander', a song John Spillane wrote for his daughter. As we listened to it together I was struck by the progress we had made. There was a time in my early twenties when I had questioned whether or not I would even want him to be at my wedding, such was my hurt at the time. Now, I couldn't wait for him to walk me down the aisle.

I am so grateful that people can change, and relationships too. I'm grateful that I can let go of old hurt and embrace new connections. I couldn't be without my dad and, even though the journey was painful at times, the result is beautiful. I am so proud of him and the work he has done to make a better life for himself and, as a result, for the rest of our family. I wouldn't change him. And that is all I have to say about that.

Andrew

You may have noticed that, when describing my early years, I mention my brother Andrew a lot. That's because we were always together. In the good times, and in the bad times, we were joined at the hip. I felt an overwhelming sense of protectiveness towards him, and a definite sense of responsibility, and often, when the chips were down, he was all I had. I think I made an effort to hide some of what went on from him, and perhaps I was somewhat successful, because these days he doesn't remember much about those early days in Ireland. This makes me happy and also sad, because, where I have a few memories of Winston, I don't think he really has any.

Of course, we were typical siblings and had our sour moments. Like the time he and his pal decided to destroy my beloved perfume collection, or the time I persuaded him to confess to having stolen a packet of biscuits when, in fact, it was me who had done it. When it came to the big stuff, however, we had each other's backs. So much so that I remember being fully convinced we would one day get married. I guess in my little brain I saw couples as a boy and a girl who did things together, and that was me and Andrew, so what else was going to happen?

Sadly, our closeness didn't last.

During the year we spent in England between moving from the US to Ireland, I excelled at school. It was just one of those times when everything came together for me: I had great friends; I was the lead in the school play; my grades were excellent. Andrew, on the other hand, struggled to adjust, and his teachers were horrible about it. 'Why can't you be more like your sister?' they would ask. As a result, he got sick of hearing about me, sick of me in general. What had been normal sibling aggro became more serious. We never really came back from it.

As we got older, our relationship grew more distant, although I still have great memories of sibling activities while we were in our teens. We used to dance our way through Top Thirty hits on RTÉ2 on a weekly basis and duetted on Linkin Park's 'In the End' on our way to the school bus in the morning. Once we moved out, though, that was kind of it. We see each other at family functions, but we don't really have our own relationship.

I find it difficult and sometimes I feel angry about it. We have a lot in common but can't seem to bridge the gap. I wonder sometimes if he remembers the closeness we once had, and how much we shared. I miss it. He is the only person in the world who went through everything with me, and yet we just don't connect.

I wonder sometimes if he remembers the closeness we once had, and how much we shared. I miss it.

Sibling relationships can be hard, especially when you're constantly confronted with perfect examples of 'best buddy' brothers and sisters on TV and in the movies. In that context, I think it's easy to feel like your relationships aren't good enough, or close enough. The reality is that not every family works that way. Not all brothers and sisters get on. So, while I haven't given up, I know I can't force it either.

Sometimes, the best thing you can do is accept things for

what they are, instead of constantly wishing they were different. Other people's relationships are exactly that – other people's – and you're only ever seeing part of the picture, the part they want you to see. Behind the scenes, they could be just as messed up as you are.

8
So, now I've written a book

Fame!

I don't know about you, but I hate it when a celebrity pretends they're not famous or talented. The whole 'Little old me? Really?' bashful shite does not sit well with me. If you are successful you should, frankly, own it and be proud of it. This is probably why I loved it when the comedian Amy Schumer ribbed Ellie Goulding over such carry-on at the 2015 Glamour Awards. When accepting an award, Ellie made a big show of how nervous she was and how she really didn't belong there but her success was for 'plain girls everywhere'.

Come on, Ellie. You're a thin, blonde multi-platinum artist who has succeeded in the US as well as at home. You're fooling no one!

When Amy got on the stage, she said, 'I'm not nervous . . . I love Ellie for being, like, "Thank you for loving real people," when she's, like, a fucking supermodel . . . But I'm, like, 160 pounds right now and I can catch a dick whenever I want, that's the truth . . . Somebody on the red carpet was, like, "Do you feel, like, out of place?" and I was, like, "No, of course not, I'm very glamorous."'

I don't think she set out to make Ellie look silly but, by completely owning her shit, she did.

I say all this because, though I want to explain a little bit about what it's been like to become a somewhat public person, I don't want to come across like one of those 'Little old me?' people. I am very proud of my success, I have worked incredibly hard for it, but I don't consider myself famous, or a celebrity.

And yet I have written a book about myself, so I must be sort of famous. The whole thing just seems a little bizarre.

No one really knew who I was until the summer of 2013, when my former boss at Newstalk and iRadio, Dan Healy, became my current boss in 2fm, and managed to convince the management that I should fill in for Ryan Tubridy while he was on his holidays. Three whole hours of high-profile morning radio. The scepticism both inside and outside RTÉ was palpable. Up to that point I had been a stand-in presenter and, although I had been presenting *Weekend Breakfast* for a year, I wasn't the owner of any show. I knew what everyone was thinking: *Who the hell is this girl and why is she getting this chance?*

The thing was, I knew I could do it and, fortunately, so did Dan. In the station, I had a meeting with two senior producers. Technically, the meeting was to discuss what kind of topics we might cover on the show during my two-week stint, but I knew what was really going on. This was my opportunity to sell myself and get these people believing in me. It would have been awful to head into that opportunity without feeling they thought I was up to it. I started the meeting by acknowledging the elephant in the room. 'So,' I said, 'I might as well say what everyone is thinking: Who the hell am I, and why is an unknown like me getting this shot?'

The producers laughed and one of them made an attempt to suggest that this was not the case, but I interrupted him. 'It's okay! It's totally understandable that you think that. It's totally understandable that people will feel that way. However, I promise you I can do this. I promise.' The tension in the room reduced somewhat, and I reeled off a long list of ideas I'd prepared of what we could do on the show while I filled in. By the end of the meeting I felt like I had them onside.

It's difficult for me to write about this without feeling an urge to downplay my confidence. However, I'm going to resist it. I *was* confident. There are loads of things I'm terrible at, but I knew I could do this.

It was during this time that I had my first dealings with newspaper reporters. Their questions were all the same. 'Were you shocked to get this opportunity?' they asked, clearly shocked themselves.

Absolutely, I told them. I had always dreamed of presenting a show like this but never really thought I would get the chance.

'Are you nervous?' they asked. The first time I was asked this question I found myself pausing, unsure of what to say. Part of me felt like I should lie and do the 'Little old me' routine, but it wouldn't have been the truth. I decided to be honest.

'No,' I told them. 'I'm not. I really believe I can do this.'

During that stint, and briefly afterwards, there were a few pieces in the paper, and subsequently when I filled in for Ryan there would often be a small bit of publicity, but that was about the extent of the media's interest in me. I didn't get invited to the fancy parties or sent stuff, like my colleagues. No one really had an interest in me. That all changed when I got cancer.

I didn't get invited to the fancy parties or sent stuff, like my colleagues. No one really had an interest in me. That all changed when I got cancer.

There was no point in keeping my diagnosis a secret. I decided to be open about it and, after speaking with Dan, it seemed that the best way to do this would be to have a chat with Ryan Tubridy on his show. If this was going to be a story, it might as well be 2fm's story. And so, about a week after being diagnosed, I went into the studio to be on the show I had been presenting a few weeks previously.

My phone blew up afterwards. Hundreds of people on Twitter sent messages of support. There were stories about me up on every Irish news website within minutes. It was weird, but also nice to see people's kindness. That was apart from one tweet – since deleted, so I can't remember the exact words – along the lines that some people had 'real cancer' and were 'really suffering' and not just looking for attention.

I cried. I cried off the eyelashes a make-up artist had applied at a magazine photoshoot I'd done two days previously. Then I cried over that. I cried because what he had said touched a nerve. I knew how lucky I was. I knew that the cancer experience I was having was not the same as the one many people go through. I knew that I had an 'easy' cancer, and in a way I felt guilty about being on the receiving end of so much kindness and interest when I knew I wasn't having the difficult time lots of cancer patients have.

The day before, I had sat in treatment with a tiny bald woman who had struggled to get the breath to talk to me but talked to me nonetheless. She had heard a nurse asking me about my wedding plans and wanted to know more. She said, 'Good, you have that to keep you going. And I have my kids.' She told me about her children and how much she loved them, and how frustrating she found it not being able to follow her usual routine at home. She'd had her eleven-year-old push her around in the wheelchair while she held the mop the previous week and sworn him to secrecy so his dad wouldn't find out. She was raging that his school had called about something and asked for her husband instead of her. They thought she'd want a break, but a break was the last thing she wanted. She was sick, properly sick, and I had walked myself to treatment that morning. I knew I was lucky.

I also cried as I tried to figure out what was happening to my life. What was I at, doing magazine photoshoots? Maybe I *was* just looking for attention?

I still haven't entirely come to terms with this. My job is in broadcasting and it's an unstated but understood part of the job description to develop a profile. To succeed, I need to be relatively well-known and to have a public persona. However, making an effort to become well-known doesn't sit comfortably with me. 'Attention-seeking' is the last phrase I would like anyone to use of me, and yet if I'm not seeking attention and trying to raise my profile and, hopefully, attract listeners, I'm not doing my job. Radio stations (and their advertisers) don't need shy, self-effacing presenters.

From early on when doing publicity, even before the cancer, I was open about many elements of my life. My American accent inevitably led to questions about my background, and I was honest about the family situation that led to me living in America for eight years. My motivation was a wish to help people who found themselves in similar situations, as I had been helped. In some ways, I was seeking attention, but for the right reasons, I hoped.

Also, a part of me is irritated for thinking that attention-seeking is the worst thing I could be. Obviously, no one likes a person who wants everything to be about them all the time, but is it so bad to ask for a little pat on the back when you've done something you're proud of? Is it bad to dye your hair a crazy colour and enjoy the reaction? Is it unforgivable to tell people you won that 5K you competed in at the weekend? Should you be silent when you're delighted about your recent promotion?

In our culture – and I think it is partly an Irish thing – we tend to avoid highlighting our achievements in order to avoid a slagging. But perhaps we could be proud of ourselves, enjoy a good-natured slagging and let that be the end of it. Maybe we could walk away from such an exchange without being afraid that people are whispering about our 'notions' or 'delusions of grandeur'. It should be okay to be proud of yourself. After all, it's not like we don't know how to wallow in self-loathing and shame when we fail. We are very good at that.

> *It should be okay to be proud of yourself. After all, it's not like we don't know how to wallow in self-loathing and shame when we fail.*

People ask me all the time what it's like being 'famous'. Well, one of the downsides of being recognizable is that you start to become a little self-conscious. Since the documentary went out in September 2015, more and more people recognize me when I'm out. People approach me on a regular basis to say hello. For the most part, it's lovely. Often they want to share an experience they've had with cancer, or just to say they've enjoyed the programme. I really like meeting them.

Occasionally, it's a bit weird – like the time I was standing on a crowded bus and the woman beside me turned to me and asked if I was Louise McSharry. I said I was and smiled, thinking this was the start of a conversation, but she just nodded and remained silent. Not going to lie: the rest of that bus journey was more than a little awkward as I stood pressed against her, struggling to maintain my balance.

The thing about these encounters is that sometimes people ask you if you're you, and then, when you say you are, they panic. Then you panic, because you don't want them to be uncomfortable, so you end up babbling like an eejit, thinking, *Please don't go away unhappy from this encounter. Please don't tell your friends I'm mean.* You start to think about how other people see you, and what stories people might tell their friends about you. 'You know that 2fm wan Louise McSharry with the cancer? I saw her on the bus the other day and she bumped into an old lady and didn't apologize.'

You find that, when you're out, the longer the night goes on and the drunker people get, the more of them come over to say hello. That's fine, but it makes you wonder if there are people spotting you when they're sober and not saying anything. And that makes you wonder if you've done anything embarrassing over the course of the night. You've seen your friends delight in telling people that a random celeb they met was a jerk. You don't want to be that jerk. You start to become very aware of how you might be coming across. You tell yourself to be careful not to get too drunk in public, because what if someone sees you and tells everyone they know that you're a mess? You tell yourself to get a grip, because no one cares. Then someone tells you that their aunty saw you on that flight to London last week and you were looking very well. *Were* you looking very well? Were you speaking too loudly? Did you say anything bad? Cop yourself on: sure, who would be listening to you? You're getting far too big for your boots. The cycle goes on.

I feel very lucky to have the opportunities I have, and I have made a choice to be a public person. I am always happy to chat to people. I feel grateful that many people feel they can share their experiences with me. But sometimes I feel a little self-conscious. I have to watch what I say when I'm in public. I can't be mean on Twitter any more. It takes some getting used to the fact that what seems like a funny, or cheeky, or ranty tweet to your community of like-minded followers can be taken out of context and turned into a story. (For the first time, on a very small scale, I understand why so many celebrities seem so boring online.) So you learn to edit what you say publicly. Still, small sacrifices.

As we know, the anonymity of the internet has made some people mean. I've been lucky, because I'm not properly famous, but lots of Irish celebs have left Twitter because they couldn't deal with the abuse. Those who go on the attack seem not to grasp that people in the media are real people with real feelings. They were real people before they were famous, and they're real people now. Famous people are human too.

I don't know if I'll become 'more famous'. That's not my goal. My aim has always been to be a successful radio presenter. I want to use whatever profile I have to draw attention to things I feel can be improved. I want to share my experiences so other people will feel less alone. I want to achieve something good in my life. And, with my skills, the more 'famous' I am, the better I can do that, I imagine. So if I become successful in the way that I want to, doing the kind of show I want to do, I probably will become better known in Ireland.

But the idea of being properly famous terrifies me. I want to be able to go to the shop in my pyjamas and clear the deli out of beige food without thinking someone's going to go home and text their mates that they saw me looking a state. I want to be able to gain and lose weight without there being commentary on it. I want to be able to wear an outfit on a night out without a celebrity website asking its readers to give it the thumbs-up or the thumbs-down!

Three things I've learned

Here's the truth. It is very hard to consider yourself in any way brave and inspirational when you know you're spending at least sixty-five per cent of your life in your pyjamas watching reality television programmes on your laptop. This was the true situation when people on Twitter were telling me I was brilliant and the newspapers started calling me a 'brave 2fm presenter'. It was all very kind, obviously, but I felt like a total fraud. All right, I had cancer, but the thing is I have always spent a fair amount of time in my pyjamas looking at my laptop.

I am a lazy person. I hate doing things unless they involve sitting down, and while I appreciate the feeling of a clean house or a freshly changed bed and the taste of a carefully cooked meal, I can rarely be bothered to make them happen myself. For that reason, my instinct is often to say no to things I should say yes to. Writing a book, for example.

People had been telling me I should write a book for years, thanks to my dramatic childhood. I always laughed off the suggestion when I was younger, but when it came from an actual person in the publishing industry I had to take it seriously. I realized I owed it to myself to give it a go.

But when I set out to write this book, I was terrified. I didn't know if I could do it, and would anyone even care? (That remains to be seen.) But I knew that, if I didn't try, I would spend years beating myself up because I had failed to seize this opportunity. And I couldn't face that. I have enough things to annoy myself with while trying to go to sleep on Sunday nights.

This is not a self-help book but I hope that maybe you've got something out of reading it. I can't let you go without sharing a few crucial principles I've learned – usually the hard way – over the years. Maybe they'll ring true for you.

First, *not everything is my responsibility*. These days, people speak a lot about anxiety. Some people have genuine anxiety disorders. And then some people are like American-reality-TV stars, talking about having 'such anxiety' over whether or not their outfit for a big event is going to arrive on time. I think I probably come somewhere in the middle.

I have a tendency to worry about things excessively, particularly about other people's happiness. I think this is a relatively normal trait for children of alcoholics to have. Years of trying to keep the peace at home and maintain some sense of normality in the family have had a lasting impact and I often find myself on alert for the next thing that's going to go wrong. I worry about whether or not other people are comfortable or if I've upset them. I convince myself sometimes that people are angry with me when they absolutely are not and I've done nothing wrong.

I hate being late, for fear that someone will be annoyed, even if it's just the hostess at a restaurant who is so used to people being late she finds my profuse apology when I am five minutes behind time bizarre. If someone is broke, I will buy them drinks because it's easier than sitting there with an overwhelming sense of empathy and concern, even though they may be perfectly happy having a night off the sauce. I have an intense feeling of concern about everyone around me, and at times it is absolutely crippling. However, it doesn't need to be that way, so I'm working on it.

Not everything is my fault. Not everything is my responsibility. It's not my job to make sure that everyone is okay at all times. My main responsibility is myself.

Second, *learning to be able to be happy for other people is one of the best things you can do for yourself.* I spent a long time in a bad place. A place of unhappiness and dissatisfaction. Things weren't going the way I wanted them to and every time I saw someone succeed in something I thought I'd be able to do I felt bitter and envious. I would be consumed with negative thoughts about their abilities, while a nasty voice in my head told me I'd be so much better than they were, if only someone would give me a chance.

Having been an overachiever for much of my life in school and at the beginning of my career in media, I couldn't understand why I had reached a time in my life when I wasn't being given a chance. Where were my opportunities? Why weren't things falling into my lap the way they were for other people? I wasted so much time and energy on this way of thinking that it pains me now. I was missing the point entirely.

Opportunities don't fall into people's laps. In fact, very little in this life just comes to you. If you want something, you have to demand it. And that's the third lesson: *you have to ask for what you want in life; otherwise, it's not going to happen.* You won't always get it right away but, if you really want it and you really think it's what's right for you, persevere.

Chances are, the bitterness you feel about other people's achievements is actually annoyance with yourself. It was certainly that way for me. I was projecting my disappointment at not having made enough of an effort to make things happen for myself on to other people. Instead of saying, 'I should really make more of an effort to make this happen,' I would say, 'Why isn't that happening to me? I deserve that!'

The thing is, once you start making things happen for yourself, you find you *are* able to be happy for other people. And it feels great. Honestly, it feels wonderful. It's a feeling so special that Buddhists have a word for it: *mudita*. They define *mudita* as 'sympathetic, vicarious joy; happiness rather than resentment at someone else's well-being or good fortune; the opposite of *schadenfreude*'.

And yes, they have a word for the feeling of resentment, too. It just goes to show you that we are not the only ones who experience it, so don't beat yourself up over it.

Afterword

In late 2015, Dee was diagnosed with lung cancer. When she started chemotherapy, she seemed positive about her prognosis. However, her body did not respond well to the treatment and she was admitted to intensive care in Northwestern Memorial Hospital in Chicago.

Initially, I did not know how to feel, or what to feel. While writing this book I had spent a good chunk of 2015 thinking about Dee and our history and, as you have read, my conclusion was that this aspect of my life wasn't something I was able to work through right now, but maybe I would someday. Now Dee was sick, and I was bewildered. I did my best to shove any thoughts about her cancer, and what it meant, to one side. I succeeded for about a week until I found myself sobbing helplessly during the show one night and I realized that maybe I had more feelings about her than I wanted to acknowledge. That night, Gordon and I booked flights and, two days later, we were in Chicago.

In her phone calls with them, my aunt told hospital staff that 'Dee's daughter' was travelling from Dublin and, when I got to Chicago, I somewhat awkwardly introduced myself that way. There was no other way to do it, really. For the first time since my childhood, I was claiming Dee.

When we got there, Dee's condition improved dramatically. She was taken off the ventilator and was able to speak again. She even sent Gordon out to get something to eat. While he was gone, I told her that writing the book had brought up a lot of intense emotion about the past and our relationship, and that I was still trying to figure things out, but that I cared about her a lot and that's why I had come.

Gordon and I spent three days in Chicago and, when we said goodbye to Dee, it was pleasant and cheerful: she was on the mend, and I had talked to her honestly about my feelings. As I left Chicago, my sense was that maybe I would be able to get a handle on how I felt about her before too long and that we would develop an easier relationship.

Unfortunately, the picture Dee had given us of her diagnosis was not accurate and the cancer was more advanced that she had first indicated. A month later – in mid-January – we were back in Chicago. Her condition had deteriorated and, during a visit from my aunt, the end seemed to be near. Andrew, my dad, my uncle, cousins, and Gordon and I, dropped everything and headed to Chicago.

Suddenly, I felt under huge pressure to try to figure it all out. Where did I really stand emotionally? What could I say that would leave us both with some peace?

I wasn't sure I'd be good at the caring bit. I've always been a little uncomfortable around sick people. It's not something I'm proud of, but I've even felt a little scared and grossed out by the physical signs of deterioration.

I needn't have worried. Some sort of instinct kicked in and I found myself slipping into the role easily. I spent a week at Dee's bedside, speaking with her and tending to her.

We spoke openly about what was going on. She speculated about how long she had left and told me she was scared. She wondered if she would be at her own funeral. I felt privileged to be there and to share these moments with her.

After a few days, most of the family had to return home to work or school. Once things were quieter, Dee asked me about this book. I had sent her the completed manuscript, but she hadn't been able to read it. I offered to read out the sections about her while I was there. The next day, she insisted that I do so.

As soon as I started, I regretted it. It felt so wrong to read Dee an account of her shortcomings while she lay on her deathbed. Several times, I asked if I should stop, but she told me to continue. I cried throughout, but she just listened, nodding from time to time. I knew from her reaction that nothing I had written surprised her. Dee herself had told her story – our story – in a radio documentary nearly ten years earlier. She didn't spare herself in it and spelled out everything she had lost because of her alcoholism. So my version of the story made sense to her.

When I finished reading it, I apologized. She told me I didn't need to. I asked her if she felt I'd been fair and accurate, and she said I had. I apologized again.

Reading the book out loud to Dee is one of the most painful things I have ever done. But I am really glad I got to do it, because I have described my experiences, and my feelings about her and about our story, more clearly and honestly in these pages than I ever managed to do in any conversation with her.

I am grateful that I got to find some peace with Dee over the course of that week. I am glad that she gave this book her blessing and I thank her for doing so.

If there's one thing of which there is no doubt, it is that Dee is a survivor. It came as a huge surprise to her medical team that, having been given just days to live, she survived the infection and sepsis that had us rushing to see her to say our goodbyes. It did not surprise us.

The hospice team attributed her remarkable turnaround to her 'fighting spirit' and the lift she had got from the visit from our family.

As I write this, Dee is very ill. Her cancer has spread and her remaining time is short. This book will be published in two months' time, but she may not live to see its publication day.

Writing a book like this is difficult, not only in the writing itself but also in returning to old feelings and situations. What I hadn't anticipated was how complicated it would be sharing the book with my family. Naturally, no one wants to relive painful memories, or to be reminded of situations that have long since been put to bed. What's even more obvious is that when you write a memoir of sorts, it's just your perspective on the past and other people might look at things differently. But if you're the one with the profile, you get to put that perspective out there, and with a kind of 'official' stamp on it because it's between the covers of a book. With that in mind, I want to say that I am more grateful than I can express that my family have encouraged me to share my story and supported its publication, even though it's hard for them to have to think about things that happened years ago, let alone have the past shared with colleagues, casual acquaintances and people they don't even know.

There is no doubt that my family and I have faced our share of challenges over the years but, like most families, we have overcome them. I wouldn't change Ruaidhrí, Ger, Andrew, Úna and Aoife for anything. There is no other family I would ever want to bicker with, or make fun of (or go to when I need to sort out my car insurance – thanks, Ruaidhrí!).

As I get older, I want to be with my family more and more. I gather that this is entirely standard for people of my age and, truly, it is a beautiful thing. It's pretty funny, too, that, often, having spent a lot of your teens fighting with them, and your twenties thinking that there's something a bit uncool about going home to hang out, now your family are among your best friends and hanging out with them is one of your favourite things to do.

There's not a whole lot of room in a book like this for stories about sitting around the kitchen table having a laugh about coming a cropper in work; or having a row about politics or music; or slagging off each other's taste; or reminiscing about relatives, teachers, bad bosses or mad neighbours; or debating which culinary disaster of the past was truly the worst; or getting advice about handling someone who's bugging you … these and the countless other conversations that go on around our kitchen table, like everyone else's. But it's important to put it on the record that we McSharrys are as wonderfully and boringly ordinary a family as you could expect to meet.

Growing up, particularly when the going was tough, I always wanted a 'normal' and 'straightforward' family. The truth is I absolutely have one. I love them, and I treasure them, and I can't wait to see what's around the corner for us all.

Postscript

I posted this blog on 1 April:

I can honestly say that throughout my experience with cancer I only thought 'WHY ME?' one time. That moment came in the office of a fertility specialist four months after being given the all-clear. The treatment that had saved my life had also decimated my egg count. Where I should have been at 35 or 40 on the scale of being able to conceive, I was a 2. I was a 2, and I was pissed off.

The doctor tried to reassure me, explaining that there were other ways, and anyway, it might happen. He told me a few stories of women who conceived naturally despite the odds being stacked against them. I felt like telling him to fuck off. I was in a dark place.

Over the following weeks I shared the bad news with some friends, who all did their best to reassure me. Many of them had their own stories of friends of friends who surprised themselves by getting pregnant when they thought they weren't able to. I shut them down one by one. I didn't want to hear about the exceptions, because they were exceptions. I couldn't bank on being an exception when I knew the probability was that I would be the rule.

Then, a few months after we started trying, I got pregnant. We spent the seven weeks between finding out and going for a scan in total disbelief, barely telling anyone, and trying not to get our hopes up. This wasn't meant to have happened! Then, last week, we saw our baby wriggling around on a screen in The Rotunda, and now there is simply no denying it. No matter what happens now, there is a baby of our creation, and I have become the exception.

We are absolutely delighted and a little bit terrified at the prospect of becoming proper adults, but I gather that's a normal way to feel. We are also incredibly grateful that we have beaten the odds.

If you are happy for us, we are very grateful for that. If, however, due to your own circumstances, you find this news difficult, I get it. I get it, and I hope that some day soon, just when you're least expecting it, you find yourself waving a wee-covered plastic stick around with delight as I recently did.

Acknowledgements

I would like to acknowledge the following people, without whom this book would not exist:

Faith O'Grady, who listened to my very sketchy idea for what this book might be and made me feel like it was a good one. Thank you for helping me quieten my imposter syndrome and for making me feel I was worthy of even having a meeting with a literary agent.

Patricia Deevy, who is a wonder-editor and managed to encourage me throughout without ever making me feel under undue pressure. Thank you for supporting me through all the ups and downs throughout the process.

Michael McLoughlin, Cliona Lewis and the wonderful team at Penguin Ireland who made me feel at home from the very start. Thanks also to the Penguin team in London – Keith Taylor, Sara Granger, Cat Hillerton, Jess Hart for the jacket and Claire Mason for the text design. Thank you to Sarah Day for eagle-eyed copy-editing.

The countless people who offered support and encouragement along the road – I am grateful to each and every one of you, including: The Squad, Glasto and the Blow-Ins, Our Heads, Aisling McDermott, Aoife Stokes, Louise O'Neill, Una Mullally, Roz Purcell, Angela Scanlan, Róisín Ingle, The Fifth Floor Collective, my colleagues at RTÉ, all my pals on Twitter (each of whom I hope to meet IRL someday), and everyone who ever told me I should write a book. Thank you for planting the seed: I hope I haven't let you down.

ACKNOWLEDGEMENTS

Noeleen, Jane, Sinéad and all the staff of St Vincent's Ward in the Mater Hospital. Your kindness, dedication and positivity were inspirational at a time which should have been the most difficult of my life. I'll never forget it.

The Spierin family. You made me feel like part of the gang from day one and have never been anything but encouraging, no matter what madness I've brought to your door.

My extended family. Thank you all for your support throughout my life, and for encouraging me always. I am so grateful that you have given me the confidence and freedom to tell my story. I have to pay a particular tribute to my paternal grandparents, Connie and Carbery Merriman. Though they're in their eighties, Granny and Grandad are both incredibly active and still work part-time. There are few people in my life who I admire as much as them, and their resilience and commitment to living a full life, despite having encountered more than their share of heartbreak, is inspiring. I am eternally grateful for all they have done and continue to do for me. Finally, my special love and thanks to:

Sarah Harte, Fiona Hyde and Emer McLysaght, who were stalwart supports throughout the process of writing the book and indeed are stalwart supports in my life in general.

Ruaidhrí, Ger, Andrew, Úna and Aoife McSharry. Thank you all for being so generous in allowing me to share my memories and perspectives. I wouldn't change our family for anything.

Gordon Spierin, who was forced to listen to me throughout this process, and is still in my life for some reason! Thank you for your patience and encouragement, and for making me feel like I could keep going when I was starting to doubt it. And thank you for sharing your life with me.